Praise for *Farewell*

"Every human deserves dignity and peace in the final chapter of life. Written by a caring physician with experience in palliative care and deep knowledge of the dying process, *Farewell* is a must-read book that could help each of us personally and also benefit those caring for the terminally ill."

Deepak Chopra, MD, FACP
Cofounder, Chopra Center for Wellbeing

"Where do you go to learn how to make a positive difference when someone you know is dying? Death is shrouded in mystery. The fear of making things worse rather than better keeps many people at a distance when they want to make a meaningful connection. The authors of this excellent book, *Farewell*, demystify the dying process. You will take away information and insights so that you can be there when someone is dying."

Vicki Rackner, MD, FACS
Retired Surgeon and Clinical Instructor
University of Washington School of Medicine
Author of *Caregiving without Regrets*

"Dr. Creagan is a compassionate and experienced physician who offers patients and families not just information and knowledge, but, more importantly, a lifetime of wisdom. Skillfully written and full of personal anecdotes, *Farewell* is an essential guide to helping individuals make wise choices about living, and dying, well."

J. Keith Mansel, MD
Professor of Medicine
Director, Palliative and Supportive Care Services
University of Mississippi Medical Center

"Knowledge provides a calming power when dealing with end-of-life issues. *Farewell* respectfully and transparently provides every element individuals and families need to traverse the often complex and always emotional quagmire of death and dying. *Farewell* will guide, inform, and create a surreal peace for anyone going through the journey for themselves or someone they know. A few tears welled up reading how my brother's passing could have been handled better had I had such a great book as *Farewell* as a ready resource."

ELAINE C PEREIRA, MA, OTR/L, CDC, CDP
Certified Dementia Practitioner, Speaker, and Caregiver
Author of award-winning book, *I Will Never Forget—
A Daughter's Story of Her Mother's Arduous
and Humorous Journey through Dementia*

"Dr. Ed Creagan has been a referring physician to the Seasons Hospice for more than twenty years. As well as being a very skilled doctor, his humor and wisdom are an asset to his patients. As Dr. Creagan states in his book, *Farewell*, he has 'dedicated his life to death,' and the community of Rochester, Minnesota, is thankful for the advocacy he has provided on end-of-life care and the importance of normalizing death as a natural part of life."

BEVERLY HAYNES, BSN, RN
Executive Director, Seasons Hospice

FAREWELL

Vital End-of-Life Questions
with Candid Answers
from a Leading Palliative and Hospice Physician

Edward T. Creagan, MD

Emeritus Professor of Medical Oncology
Mayo Clinic Medical School

with SANDRA WENDEL

WRITE ON INK
PUBLISHING

Patient privacy: With medical privacy laws, which I deeply respect, and my oath as a physician to maintain privacy, I will introduce you to some of the types of people I see with dreadful diseases. Their stories, a compilation of experience and example, will serve to paint a broad picture of the end of life. Facts and details have been changed, of course, to mask identities, but each patient's story remains with me and shapes my growth as a physician and human being.

Medical disclaimer: The information contained in this book is not intended as a substitute for the advice and/or medical care of the reader's physician, nor is it meant to discourage or dissuade the reader from seeking the advice of his or her physician. If the reader has any questions concerning the information presented in this book, or its application to his or her particular medical profile or the medical profile of a family member or friend at the end of life, he or she should consult his or her physician and the attending physicians of the ill person. Neither the authors nor the publisher shall be liable or responsible for any loss or damage allegedly arising as a consequence of the reader's use or application of any information or suggestions in this book.

This book reflects the individual views and opinions of Edward T. Creagan, MD.

Library of Congress Cataloging Number: 2018952652
Cataloging-in-Publication Data on file with publisher.

Paperback ISBN: 978-0-9916544-8-2
Kindle ISBN: 978-0-9916544-9-9
EPUB ISBN: 978-1-7326404-1-2
Audiobook ISBN: 978-1-7326404-2-9

Write On Ink Publishing
Omaha, Nebraska
(402) 334-2547
Publisher@Q.com

Contact the author for speaking engagements and events through the publisher or www.AskDoctorEd.com.

TO THE PATIENTS AND FAMILIES
who have shared their stories of courage,
tenacity, and grace at the end of life.

CONTENTS

INTRODUCTION xi
How to Use This Book at the Bedside

1. **How Can We Die a Good Death?** 1
What I've Learned at the Bedside

2. **What Happens at the Deathbed?** 7

3. **What Is Death, Actually?** 15
Keeping Someone Alive
(but Are They Really Living?)
Tying Up Loose Ends
The Process of Dying
Quality of Life and Death
Respect for Cultural Beliefs

4. **Don't We Have the Right to Die?** 29
Dying on Your Own Terms

5. **Why Does a Person's Life Story
Matter at the End of Life?** 33

6. **What Do We Do When the Doctor
Delivers Bad News?** 41

7. **"Doc, How Long Do I Have to Live?"** 47
The Problem with Optimism
"What Would You Do, Doc?"

8. **May I Share My Story about Palliative Care?** 57

9. **How Does Palliative Care Fit?** 63
How and When to Get a Palliative Consult
Palliative Care at the End of Life

10. **How Did Palliative Care and Hospice
Evolve to Become Such Key Components
of End-of-Life Care?** 75
A Brief History
The Medicare Hospice Benefit

Getting Answers to Hard Questions
Capacity versus Competence

11. **What Is Hospice?**............................89
Types of Hospice Settings
And Now a Little Insight

12. **Why Is the Family Meeting So
Critically Important?**.......................95
What Happens When the Family Cannot Agree?
When Hospice Might Be Considered

13. **What Is Patient-Centered Management
at the End of Life?**.........................107
The Empowered Patient, the Informed Family
There's Always Hope

14. **When Do We Start and Stop Medication?**.....115

15. **How Can We Relieve Pain?**..................119
The Three-Step Approach to Treating Pain
Controlling Side Effects of Pain Medications
What about Addiction?
Intractable Pain
Steroids
Antidepressants
Alternative Medicine

16. **How Do We Control Other Symptoms?**.......133
Fear of Suffocation, Shortness of Breath
Inability to Swallow, Fear of Choking
Lack of Appetite, Weight Loss
Incontinence
Inability to Speak
Fatigue
Nausea and Vomiting
Bowel Obstruction

Delirium, Confusion
Lack of Sleep

17. **How Do Doctors Manage the Diseases of Death?**..........................143
Congestive Heart Failure
Dementia
Chronic Obstructive
Pulmonary Disease (COPD)

18. **What Does "Do Not Resuscitate" (DNR) Really Mean?**........................151

19. **How Do We Make Sense of Deathbed Confessions?**..............................155
How to Start the Bedside Conversation
What Dying People Say and Why They Say It
Greed (or Who Gets What)—
Plain and Not So Simple

20. **Who Pulls the Plug?**.........................165
When the Plug Is Pulled

21. **How Do We Resolve Ethical Dilemmas in Decision-Making for the Dying? The Role of the Advance Directive and Healthcare Proxy** ...173
The Advance Directive
A Partnership with Patient Rights and
Caregiver Responsibilities
The Needs of the Patient Come First
Responsibilities and Fears of the
Healthcare Surrogate

22. **Can You Help Me Understand the Advance Directive?** 185

23. **Who Are the Players around the Bed?** 191
The Family Doc

The Insurance Company
An Outside Caregiver
The Unwanted Visitor (Virtually and Otherwise)

24. **What about Physician-Assisted Suicide?** 199

25. **How Do We Help in Grieving**
    for Life and Loss?..........................205
    The Myth of Not Battling Hard Enough
    Pain of the Soul
    Spirituality and Religion
    Glass Half Full?
    Grief in the Survivors

26. **Who Cares for the Caregivers?** 219
    Caring for Yourself
    How Palliative and Hospice Care
        Benefit the Caregiver

27. **What If the Doctors Ask about an Autopsy?**....227
    Organ Donation

28. **How Do We Plan for the Funeral?**.............231

29. **Has Anyone Considered the Cost of Dying?**....235

30. **What Is the Role of Complementary**
    and Alternative Medicine at the End of Life? ...239

31. **What Lessons Have We Learned?** 243

RESOURCES 249

ACKNOWLEDGMENTS.........................251

INDEX 255

ABOUT THE AUTHORS 259

INTRODUCTION

I have dedicated my life to death.

For over forty winters at the Mayo Clinic in Rochester, Minnesota, I have been at the bedside with more than 40,000 patient encounters in the last stages of their lives on this earth. Held the hands of family members. Prayed with them. Listened. Answered questions (not all questions had answers, such as these: *How long am I going to live? Who will be with me? Will my family forgive me?* and *Will I have pain?*).

This book is about navigating those last days and saying farewell with hope, love, and compassion.

About making end-of-life decisions when Mom or Dad or a loved one can't or won't.

About understanding what's happening in the mind of someone facing their last days, hours, minutes, and moments.

About coming to grips with our own mortality, maybe putting plans in place, living life differently after having held the hand of a loved one who is actively dying.

About giving hope where none seemed possible.

About understanding death from a medical perspective, and much more.

I am trained as an oncologist, a cancer specialist. Heart disease is the leading cause of death, but cancer is the most feared. Patients would rather be told their heart muscle is failing than that they have a mass in their pancreas or liver or lung or breast.

Many cancer patients are cured and go on to live a long and healthy life. Others are not so fortunate. I'm sorry to tell this to former Vice President Joe Biden, who was charged with advancing cancer treatment and cure, but the war on cancer—begun with legislation and research funds back in the Nixon administration—remains a multifront battle. Yes, it has seen some exciting progress here and there, but, because cancer comprises many diseases, we will continue to fight it for a very long time.

When we cancer doctors—and especially in my practice at Mayo Clinic—see patients with far-advanced disease, the treatment we offer them is often comfort and dignity and choice and hope. No magic bullets. No miracle potions.

As our patients face their own death, we extend our care to them in practices called *palliative care* (a medical specialty known for managing symptoms and providing comfort measures) and *hospice* (for patients who are assessed to have just months to live and are not pursuing treatment for their terminal illness). Of course, we are happily surprised when someone rallies for reasons beyond the understanding of modern medicine, but often the road leads to a bedside and family members gathered around, consoling, cajoling, and saying farewell.

I have board certification in internal medicine, medical oncology, and palliative and hospice medicine. I was the first Mayo Clinic doctor certified in this specialty, and I am grateful to the thousands of patients and their families and loved ones who allowed me to take their final journeys with them. I have now stepped away from active clinical practice and leave as my legacy this book that sums up my years of experience with families just like yours.

This is a book about the end of life. Boomers are saying goodbye to their parents and facing their own mortality. In a perfect world, we live a long life and then die. No sickness. No suffering. It's called compression of morbidity—meaning we live life to its fullest, without illness or pain, and simply slip away in our sleep.

Death doesn't often happen that way.

I'm not talking about tragic accidents that cut short young lives or any lives. I refer to long, protracted illness, loss of the abilities to just, well, live or live well—when decisions need to be made about care, levels of care, where care is to be done, and guesses are made about life expectancy, and days are measured in days remaining.

Illness tears families apart, not only emotionally but financially and geographically. Sometimes fences don't get mended. The prodigal son may not return. Past regrets surface. At the bedside, patients and their families may reach a new normal as life goes on without a member at the table, yet life is never quite the same.

Before I explain what this book is, let me tell you what this book is not.

It is not a history of hospice. If you want to learn about that, read *Hospice and Palliative Medicine Handbook: A Clinical Guide* by Susan Bodtke, MD, and Kathy Ligon, MD.

It is not a how-to on dealing with a terminal diagnosis or coming to terms with death. If you want to read a poignant treatise on how to face death and life with a terminal diagnosis, read Professor Randy Pausch's *The Last Lecture*—a classic. Another unforgettable reflection on facing death is Dr. Paul Kalanithi's *When Breath Becomes Air.* He became both patient and doctor.

It is not an existential assessment of life from the perspective of a physician. I wish I were talented enough to have written this book—*Being Mortal: Medicine and What Matters in the End*—but Dr. Atul Gawande already did.

I have attempted to fill a different niche with this book. This is the information I hope you may find helpful before you need to make decisions about stopping Dad's chemotherapy or whether to see if he can endure yet another surgery; or if Mom should die in a nursing home or be brought home and surrounded with family and love; or whether Aunt Bea is capable of deciding whether she should have a feeding tube or if cousin Frank can make that decision (or even should); or any number of decisions surrounding the bedside at the end of life.

First Lady Barbara Bush made her decision to stop active treatment in and out of hospitals and went home surrounded by her loving family where she received comfort care until her death. These brave and loving scenarios are playing out in homes and with families every day.

During the writing of this book, we talked with people just like you. Their bedside experiences were often fresh in their memories, even if their loved one had died years ago. They told us their stories, and we have included some of their wisdom here. To them, we are indeed grateful.

Sadly, many of you may be reading this book because you are sitting at the bedside of a loved one whose health is declining. You are in the eye of the medical storm. I hope my words will give you the type of hope I have given to thousands of families and patients over the years. I don't know you, but I know where you are and the questions you need answers to.

So let's get started.

How to Use This Book at the Bedside

I know that family members in crisis situations don't sit down and read a book like this cover to cover. You can't. You're distracted. You're emotionally and spiritually drained. You face an uncertain future, and you're being asked to make life-and-death decisions.

Our test readers often told us, "I wish I had this book when I was sitting by my mother's bed." We have organized the book to answer the most pressing questions you may have. Use the table of contents to find the sections most relevant to you. I have repeated some of the material from time to time because I know you won't read everything, and I've commented to let you know this so that you can explore topics more deeply if desired. And we have created a helpful, easy-to-use index at the back of the book to guide your more in-depth search for information and understanding.

My coauthor and I welcome your feedback at the book's website (*www.AskDoctorEd.com*) so we can incorporate your thoughts and suggestions in the next version for the next family facing the same journeys you are taking.

I wish you well.

1

How Can We Die a Good Death?

THE PHONE CALL CAME EARLY ON A SUNDAY MORNING, ON A bitterly cold February day in 1992. That phone call forever changed the direction of my professional life. On the end of the line was Willie, my mother's second husband. Willie was part of the Greatest Generation that fought in some of the bloodiest battles of World War II. He was involved in the tank battles of North Africa, as well as the invasion of Italy in the battles of Monte Cassino and Anzio. Like many returning veterans, he never really talked about these experiences.

Willie was a high school dropout; he was a good person. He scraped together a few bucks and bought a bar and two liquor stores in Newark, New Jersey. I therefore spent a lot of my formative years "behind bars."

Following the death of my mother from breast cancer and alcoholism in the 1980s, Willie and I drifted apart. We were never close to begin with. He was a blue-collar guy—shots and a beer, and flannel shirts—whereas I was more focused on academic and scholarly activities. We exchanged the obligatory phone calls on Father's Day and at Christmas, but our worlds were very different.

When that Sunday-morning phone call came, it was obvious that Willie was sick. He had been a heavy smoker and a heavy drinker, and over the phone he was clearly hoarse, short of breath, obviously weak—and terrified. When he told me about the blood in the phlegm he was hacking up, my concern was lung cancer.

Willie came to see me at Mayo Clinic, where I was a cancer specialist. On the morning of surgery an incision was made behind the breastbone to analyze the lymph nodes. If these lymph nodes did not have cancer, Willie's lung would be removed with a hope of a cure. But let me tell you what happened.

About twenty minutes into the procedure, I received a phone call from the surgical dispatch nurse that the surgeon wanted to meet me. This was not good news. If the lung had been removed, that would have been a four-hour procedure. I remember the encounter as if it happened yesterday.

In the midst of a busy clinical ward surrounded by medical teams making rounds, the surgeon greeted me. He was gloved, gowned, and masked, making it difficult to decipher what he had to say. But I did manage to make out his critical comments: "The nodes are full of cancer. There's nothing we can do."

I felt stunned, overwhelmed, paralyzed. Even though I had been a cancer doctor for more than twenty years, I was completely blindsided by this encounter. After I collected my thoughts and absorbed the magnitude of the news, Willie and I met. We hugged, we cried, and we tried to plan out the future.

I will not explain in detail how this experience unfolded, but it was the first time I so deeply recognized that there had to be a more compassionate way to share bad news and to enhance the quality of life for patients and families during one of the most difficult times in their lives.

The last several months of Willie's life were not pretty. He had every symptom imaginable from his lung cancer. He was short of breath. He was in pain. He was constipated. He was not sleeping. He had overwhelming anxiety. He also suffered from a type of spiritual distress that is also called an existential crisis. Very simply, this meant he was asking the big questions: *What is life all about? Does my life have meaning, purpose, and engagement?*

Will I leave any sort of legacy? There was no expression of love or forgiveness. There was no attempt to mend fences or close painful chapters.

Now, I want to be perfectly honest and in no way critical. In the early 1990s there was little recognition of the spiritual factors in the quality of life for cancer patients. There was little concept of hospice at that time in the medical world, and Willie languished in a local hospital for several months. We whisked him to the intensive care unit from time to time as conditions worsened. Ultimately, he died, an angry, bitter, disenfranchised individual.

This was hardly the "good death" that we sometimes read about. The typical obituary often describes the patient dying at home, without pain and in peace, surrounded by a loving, adoring family. The patient slips into sleep to receive his or her reward in the next life. This is the kind of death we all fantasize about, but death doesn't always happen quite so neatly.

Let me explain. Based on studies by researchers from various institutions, including the National Institute on Aging, people dying of cancer were highly functional (could take care of themselves, dress, bathe, and eat, for example) early in the final year of life but became more disabled three months before death. Patients suffering from organ failure, such as from heart disease, fluctuated in their decline but showed great disability in the three months before death. And our frail elderly showed marked decline in the last year of life, in and out of the hospital, with intense dependence on caregivers during the last month of life.

My colleagues in palliative care at the Veterans Affairs Medical Center in North Carolina and elsewhere conducted a landmark study by asking patients, their family members, doctors, and healthcare providers what they considered important at the end of life. The results were in the *Journal of the American Medical Association*.

Pain and symptom management remain paramount, as does communicating with the doctor, preparing for death, and having the opportunity to achieve a sense of completion and/or closure. Other issues were rated "important" by more than 70 percent of the participants in the study. Think about what you consider important as you read this list from the study:

- Be kept clean
- Name a decision-maker
- Have a nurse with whom one feels comfortable
- Know what to expect about one's physical condition
- Have someone who will listen
- Maintain one's dignity
- Trust one's physician
- Have financial affairs in order
- Be free of pain
- Maintain sense of humor
- Say goodbye to important people
- Be free of shortness of breath
- Be free of anxiety
- Have physician with whom one can discuss fears
- Have physician who knows one as a whole person
- Resolve unfinished business with family or friends
- Have physical touch
- Know that one's physician is comfortable talking about death and dying
- Share time with close friends
- Believe family is prepared for one's death
- Feel prepared to die
- Presence of family
- Treatment preferences in writing
- Not die alone
- Remember personal accomplishments
- Receive care from personal physician

Similarly, researchers at the University of California, San Diego School of Medicine completed a literature search defining a "good death." After interviews with patients, family members, and healthcare providers, they identified these eleven themes:

- Preferences for a specific dying process
- Pain-free status
- Religiosity/spirituality
- Emotional well-being
- Life completion
- Treatment preferences
- Dignity
- Family
- Quality of life
- Relationship with the healthcare provider
- Other

The findings are in the *American Journal of Geriatric Psychiatry*.

The researchers offered this advice, and I concur because I do this at the bedside: Ask the patient what is important to them in order to have a good death. And then do your best to make that happen. I think it is reasonable for family members to ask their loved one that same question: What are you most concerned about?

What I've Learned at the Bedside

Willie's experience opened the door, and opened my mind, in terms of a better way to navigate the end of life. Throughout the pages of this book I will share with you what I've learned from my own experiences and what I've learned from other professionals dealing in a complex area of medicine where there is a murky interface between law and ethics and medical care—a place where the rules are sometimes blurry, a place where decisions are often made based upon ethical and religious and spiritual dimensions, a place where we can make a difference in the quality of life for patients and families. For only then can we bid a fond farewell and know that it truly is.

2
What Happens at the Deathbed?

"I HAD BEEN SLEEPING IN A CHAIR NEXT TO THE COUCH WHERE my sister was dying, at home, surrounded by her dogs. Five tiny Chihuahuas were curled up with her, around her legs and on her shoulder. She hadn't spoken for several hours now. It was day four." These are the recollections of my coauthor, whose sister was actively dying from tracheal cancer at age sixty-four.

12:30 a.m., March 31

"I was startled awake by a rasping sound, a struggled breathing, so I searched Google on my iPad for *death rattle*. Yes, that's what I was hearing. My sister was unable to speak now. She had slipped into a deep sleep. We had given her the regularly scheduled dose of morphine and lorazepam earlier.

"I called the hospice. They confirmed that I had heard the death rattle and directed me to the package of emergency medicine they had placed in the refrigerator. I don't recall what the medication was, but it was a dropper of medicine to dry up her throat secretions. We had taken away the oxygen hours earlier. The hospice people, in one of my many phone calls that day, said it was no longer of value."

2:45 a.m., March 31

"In the flickering light of the TV, which we had kept on more for comfort of sound and light than enlightenment of world events, I roused and heard it. Silence. No death rattle. No strug-gled breathing. And the dogs had instinctively moved from the couch to chairs around the room. Their work was done. My sister had died. I felt profoundly calm, relieved actually, that she was no longer suffering. And great sadness."

Many of us never see the dying process. Historically in an agrarian society, farm animals would be born and would die, and the life-and-death cycle was familiar to everyone. Today, this is not the case.

We need to recognize that someone who is dying is sur-rounded in an envelope of losses: physical and cognitive losses, social and emotional losses, and also a spiritual loss that calls into question their faith or belief system.

Let me walk you through the dying process so that there is some understanding of what to expect.

Although there are wide variations in people and circum-stances, most of us—approximately 85 percent—will die from a prolonged, ongoing process. However, during the terminal events, there are fairly predictable signs that death is imminent. And this can be of great comfort to families, as it provides a general timetable of what is happening.

For most families, the death of a spouse, a partner, or a family member—if guided with kindness, compassion, and forethought—can be a time of great enrichment.

Clinically speaking, there are some fairly predictable phases of dying. These are initially characterized by accelerating fatigue, weakness, and increased time sleeping. A loved one may become less engaged in conversations. They become easily distracted and spend far more time in a semivegetative state where arousal may be difficult.

As this process continues over a number of hours or days, they may become confused. They may also demonstrate a blue discoloration of the hands and feet, an inability to close their eyes, and difficulty closing their mouth, which may remain open. These clinical predictions aside, the transition from life to death is a sacred passage, and honoring it with dignity, grace, mercy, and love can provide enrichment—emotionally, psychologically, and spiritually. This applies throughout all phases of the dying process, as the sacred so often is the element in control, mystifying and humbling all present, including us doctors.

Returning to our clinical discussion, once someone enters into the active process of dying, survival is usually limited to about one to two weeks, although this number can be highly variable. Many people become completely exhausted and spiritually spent. Many will stop eating and drinking. At that point, survival may be eight to ten days, but for a well-nourished and relatively young person, the time until death may be longer.

So what typically happens during this dying process?

Approximately half of people dying will develop a noisy, gurgling sound that is often called the death rattle (as described my coauthor's reflection of her sister's process). This can be distressing to family members but, in general, is of little significance to the person. By positioning the person on one side or the other, this noise can commonly be decreased.

The change in breathing sounds or development of the death rattle usually indicates that death will occur within about twenty-four to forty-eight hours. A number of medications can be considered to dry up secretions and perhaps lessen the sound, but, for the most part, drugs are not necessary and don't help.

A common dilemma that we doctors face is the real challenge of how to advise family members who live at a great distance from where the person is dying. In general, one philosophy is to encourage the family member to travel to the bedside within a reasonable period of time. As the days evolve, people who are dying become more confused and less conversant, and the important work of mending fences and making amends can only be done when the person can engage in conversations.

An incredible source of distress to patients and families is the waxing and waning of unconsciousness, delirium, and hallucinations. Therefore, if someone is out of town and "waiting for the final hours," consider that it would be more comforting for all if the visit came earlier rather than later.

I have seen it more often than not. The estranged son shows up just as Dad takes his final breath. No one knows how long the process of dying will take, but once someone has entered that corridor, I always stress that anyone waiting to come should do so sooner rather than later. On some occasions I have even urged that the date of a prison release or probation be moved up as a compassionate gesture so that the family member can be with the dying person. On the other end of the spectrum, I have advised moving up the dates of weddings and other celebrations so that they will precede the death event.

Urinary incontinence occurs in about one-third of people at this stage of the process. Without question, about half develop agitation, confusion, and restlessness. A common, distressing sign for families is an unpredictable jerking of arms and legs, sometimes to the point of throwing off the bedclothes. This is called myoclonus, and it's rare. It does not represent a seizure and can often reflect changes in body functioning; it is especially common when people are taking opiates such as morphine for pain.

Instead of that peaceful death described in obituaries, in a complex death, patients with myoclonus are racked by this jerking of arms and legs, and also experience uncontrollable delirium, both of which are incredibly distressing for family members. Since, in most patients, these symptoms are direct results of morphine or related pain medications, it's important for you to ask the medical team to explain this and adjust the medication.

Even though someone may be lapsing into a coma, most people (an estimated 90%) may well need continuing pain medications. If someone is unable to take medications by mouth, a drop of concentrated morphine under the tongue can be of tremendous value. Suppositories can be used, but these are often not acceptable to the patient or the family unless a healthcare professional administers them. (A suppository is placed in the rectum.)

Shortness of breath is a common concern. Although the data supporting the use of oxygen is questionable (it may not be life prolonging, and, certainly, the lack of it is not killing the patient at this stage), there can be a psychological advantage for the family. Anxiety can be the source of a tremendous acceleration of shortness of breath, and the doctor may suggest medicines such as Ativan (generic name is lorazepam) to lessen the anxiety, as well as morphine to decrease air hunger.

For reasons that are unclear, a low-speed fan directed across the patient's face can be comforting. Just think about the dog in the car who insists on sticking his muzzle out the open window. There are delicate nerve endings in the face, and exposing them to a column of air can provide a source of great comfort.

What else can we do at the bedside? Provide a lighted room. Maintain a calm atmosphere. Have familiar items at the bedside—such as photos, religious articles, a calendar, and a clock—as these can often assist. Play music. And if the patient is in a hospital or hospice setting away from home, don't overlook the person's favorite pillow or blanket, or a familiar quilt or handmade afghan.

Thirst and hunger in the patient are common concerns for caregivers. Almost never is thirst a major issue. Careful attention to mouth hygiene, with appropriate swabs, ice chips, Popsicles, and frozen, slushy Gatorade, and the use of lemon drops and related agents, can be of great comfort.

Multiple studies have confirmed that hearing is the last of the senses to fade. So we must all be aware that the dying patient who may appear to be in a coma or deep sleep may indeed hear conversation around the bedside. Be respectful and be discreet; this is not about you. In fact, in many instances, when individuals have been resuscitated, they report that they were able to hear what was going on around them.

If you feel so inclined, it's tender and calming to sit by the bedside and hold the hand of a loved one. Talk to the person and tell them how you are feeling. *(Mom, you were always there for me. I will miss you. OR, I wasn't always the best sister, but we shared so much together. You are leaving us, and we will remember your bright smile and generosity.)* This is, of course, not the time to dredge up the past. Rather, it is the time to send them off gently, with forgiveness, spoken or tacit, assuring them that it's okay to let go, that you both will be at peace.

Although we cannot accurately predict the moment of death, if the death rattle occurs (it doesn't always occur), when the person becomes more comatose, and when the extremities begin to turn blue, death will typically occur within a short number of hours or days.

Most families are completely unprepared for the flood of emotions and experiences at the actual moment of death. This is a sacred moment. It is the moment when life ceases, and it can be profoundly quiet, even mystical—or shrouded in denial.

According to Donna Miesbach, in her book, *From Grief to Joy:*

> Mother's passing was different from my two previous losses. Both my husband and my father were snatched away so suddenly. Not so with Mother. Hers was a graceful passage. We'd had the whole day together, and while she hadn't been able to say a word, words hadn't been necessary. We seemed to be enveloped in a sacred space, and we were content just to be there, to let happen what was happening. Knowing that neither of us could stop it, we were

able to accept it for what it was as she slipped into the sacred mystery we have yet to fathom.

Being present at the bedside, and even at the moment of death, can become an experience embedded in the minds and souls of family members for generations. It is a deeply emotional time, one of relief and sadness. Anyone who has taken that final journey with someone will never, ever forget those moments.

3
What Is Death, Actually?

BRIAN WAS IN A SEVERE AUTOMOBILE ACCIDENT AND SUFFERED extensive brain injury. He was sustained with artificial ventilation for breathing, artificial kidney support (dialysis), and an armada of intravenous fluids and medications to maintain his blood pressure and to control for infection. There was no reasonable probability for improvement. He was otherwise healthy at age forty-four. At what point should we consider him "dead"?

This isn't a question on a medical school exam. This is real-life drama played out every day in the emergency rooms and intensive care units (ICUs) across the country.

The usual definition of death is the cessation of biological functions that sustain a living organism. There is general agreement in medical circles that this is an appropriate definition. But with modern technology, the definition of death becomes much more complicated.

These decisions really defy a unified approach, but most medical professionals embrace some general concepts. If the individual cannot be supported without the use of these interventions, such as those sustaining Brian, and if brain wave tests indicate no active function, that patient may be declared legally dead. Life as we know it would cease if these interventions were discontinued.

The issue of brain death is racked with profound philosophical and religious implications. Brain death is often defined as the complete loss of brain function, including involuntary activity necessary to sustain life. An important distinction is that of a persistent vegetative state in which a person is "alive," and there is some autonomic function (spontaneous activity, such as breathing, controlled by the nervous system). Individuals may exist in this state for decades.

When there is great controversy about the management of these patients, it is certainly important to seek the counsel of the appropriate specialist, such as the neurologist, the palliative care consultant, and, in some cases, a medical ethics expert.

The issue of when a patient is "dead" is murky, clouded in controversy, and this can be a source of great anguish for the family and the medical team.

Historically, before the advent of modern resuscitation and technology, the patient was typically declared "dead" when the heart ceased to function. The physician would listen to the chest, and if there were no heart sounds and no pulse, the patient was deemed to have died.

However, with the use of intubation and lung support and dialysis and other supportive interventions, the issue of death can be fraught with much legal, ethical, and medical peril.

The current trend in this area is to focus on brain function. There are few, if any, exceptions of a revival of a patient following the irreversible cessation of all functions of the brain. This is typically documented by brain wave analyses in conjunction with a neurologic examination by a neurologist who has expertise in this difficult area. The presence or absence of certain reflexes, certain spontaneous signs and symptoms, would all indicate that there is no reasonable probability that the patient would survive.

We are all familiar with a rare but remarkable case where an individual was deemed to have died but was able to spontaneously recover. These are extraordinary and infrequent circumstances that really complicate this situation. There is a general consensus that legal death is determined by the irreversible stoppage of the heartbeat without spontaneously breathing and by the cessation of functions of the brain. And these are in concert with the Uniform Determination of Death Act.

Someone in authority and legal standing then pronounces a person to have died and notes the time. That someone is generally a physician in the hospital, a hospice professional (if the person dies at home or in hospice), the coroner, or any number of medical and healthcare professionals in nursing homes, even sheriffs and other members of law enforcement, depending on the laws in any given state.

Keeping Someone Alive (but Are They Really Living?)

When faced with the agonizing situation of whether to sustain an individual artificially, obviously, family members may seek the counsel of a spiritual advisor or member of leadership in a faith community, in addition to considering the advice of the medical team.

In the absence of a legal mandate, such as healthcare power of attorney, to make these crucial life-and-death decisions, family members, when faced with the question of whether to discontinue kidney dialysis or remove the respirator, often find comfort when they consider this question: If Mom could turn back the clock one hour and sit up in bed, what would she share with us about her wishes?

Most find comfort in making these hard decisions to discontinue mechanical intervention, with all of its miseries and suffering, and allow death to embrace the patient who then can die in a natural environment.

Tying Up Loose Ends

Whether it's the estate planning or repairing hurt feelings or a lifetime of envy or squabbling, tying up these loose ends is the responsibility of the family early in the course of a patient's illness. This is important because it allows that chapter to be closed. The focus can then be placed on the tasks of dying, as eloquently outlined by Dr. Ira Byock, a leading palliative physician, in his many books.

These tasks, listed here in modified form, provide families with an important guide to understanding where patients are coming from:

- **Ask for forgiveness.** This is an amazingly common phenomenon. We each have made transgressions. We each have injured others. I can recall many vivid experiences of a bedside reconciliation with family members or business partners.

- **Forgive yourself.** Dr. Byock talks about offering forgiveness, and one dimension of this that I commonly see is forgiving ourselves. An overwhelmingly high proportion of cancers are directly related to lifestyle options and lifestyle choices, such as smoking or excessive sun exposure. Equally important, most heart disease reflects behavioral choices, such as a sedentary lifestyle, a high-fat diet, and excessive stress. Almost never do I recall a patient acknowledging their role in their illness. However, when such acknowledgment does occur, it gives that patient a tremendous sense of peace and freedom.

- **Offer thanks.** Offering thanks is embedded in the soul of almost every patient. I'm often touched by the patient who will ask me how I am doing when, in fact, the patient is dealing with a terminal illness and a relatively short survival. That ability to get out of our shell and reach out, even at the end of life, can be an elixir of peace and serenity, and the task of offering expressions of love is absolutely miraculous. The touch, the hug, the note thanking family members or members of the care community is a gentle way of saying, "I fought the good fight. I'm tired. I could not have done this without each of you, and now it's time to say goodbye."

Now, we need to understand that these tasks do not evolve in a predictable pattern. Some patients, because of cultural or societal experiences, do not have the capability of expressing thanks and love. And that's okay.

Candy told me about how her dear mother kept hanging on despite the removal of all artificial nutrition and other bedside measures at home, in keeping with the family's deeply religious request for a peaceful passing. The round-the-clock nursing staff was astounded that Mama continued to hang on, day after day.

"Is there someone she's waiting for?" the nurses asked Candy.

"No, we're all here," Candy said, puzzled by what her mother might be waiting for.

After eleven days into the family vigil around the bedside, Candy's two grown children had a real knock-down, drag-out fight that evening about their contentious relationship, which had characterized their interactions all their lives. At the end was heartfelt reconciliation, and the air was cleared. Candy's mother, their grandmother, died the next morning.

No one can explain the phenomenon, but I have seen it more times than coincidence would explain. Family members reconciled, forgiveness expressed, atonement found, apologies made, secrets revealed, consciences cleared, promises made, misunderstandings resolved, grievances aired—every family has this type of baggage, and it often surfaces during end-of-life experiences, frequently leading to resolution or, at least, acceptance and peace.

I am often asked about giving someone permission to die, to let go. I am comfortable saying that, yes, some patients need to be given permission to go. You can assure your sister that she has fought the good fight and given it her best shot, that she is loved, and that you will carry out her wishes. You can quietly whisper in your mother's ear that everyone is there; it's okay to go. You can clutch your father's hand and remind him that he was strong, and now you'll be strong in his absence. Every family will find their own way to ease the passage.

The Process of Dying

The process of dying is exactly that. It is a process, an evolution, a journey. Each patient brings to the dying process a unique psychological and spiritual and physical dimension, but there are some remarkably similar characteristics. In addition, there are also some reasonably predictable physiological, biological, and medical processes that are important to understand. Let's explore the process a bit more deeply now.

Most family members have never seen someone die, so they are completely unprepared for these experiences, which can be devastating. Here's what may be helpful for families to know to help them understand what to expect as the patient's dying process unfolds.

Patients predictably have fatigue, which means that simple actions like sitting in a chair can become absolutely draining. Their attention span becomes limited because of fatigue, and we need to understand the importance of limiting encounters with the dying patient, simply because they do not have enough energy.

Patients gradually become withdrawn and have less energy for social engagements and conversation. Therefore, visitors to the patient who is dealing with a serious illness must understand how draining it is for that patient to deal with the trivial chatter of everyday life. Visitors may want to talk about the weather, news from other family members, or an upcoming high school graduation. Visitors can be uncomfortable and feel compelled to talk about something—anything.

Well, 80 percent of life is just showing up, as comedian Woody Allen said. So just show up. You don't have to say anything. Your physical presence can provide powerful sustenance during this difficult time. Save the idle chatter about football scores to share with family members in the hospital's waiting room, nursing home's hallway, hospice family waiting area, or kitchen if visiting someone at home.

Our culture revolves around meals and food. If we think about it, almost every human event of significance in our culture is associated with the barbecue, the picnic, the formal dinner, the luncheon. Families need to understand that as the dying process evolves, the drive to eat and drink becomes dramatically blunted.

Patients almost never have a desire to eat or drink, because their appetite becomes depressed and the sensation of thirst typically disappears within several days. It's important that family members understand that there is no advantage to push fluids, and there is no advantage to "force-feed" patients, since this can be disruptive.

Now let's focus just for a moment on the issue of feeding tubes. Without doubt, this controversy arises in virtually every patient, and the discussion goes something like this: "But, Doc, you can't let Mom starve to death. She'll die of dehydration or malnutrition! You have to do something."

We now know from peer-reviewed studies that there are tremendous risks with the feeding tube placed into the nose and then into the stomach, or to the feeding tube that is placed through the abdominal wall into the stomach. This is typically called a PEG tube, which stands for percutaneous endoscopic gastrostomy. A high-calorie nutritional mix is dripped through these tubes directly into the stomach.

It seems to be almost common sense that if we supply nutrition in a liquid form through these tubes, this will enhance the patient's appetite and sense of well-being and thereby improve their outcome. The reverse is the actual fact.

Multiple studies have looked at patients who've had these devices, and, overwhelmingly, their quality of life deteriorates. They have all sorts of biochemical imbalances. Many struggle with diarrhea and abdominal cramps, and some also aspirate. The latter means that oral secretions, rather than being swallowed, go down the bronchial air tube, lodge in the lungs, and cause aspiration pneumonia. One of the reasons for the development of pneumonia is that when patients have tubes, they are typically in the fetal position, lying on one side with their knees brought up to their chest—the ideal position to provoke aspiration pneumonia.

Mechanical interventions can be disastrous and do not enhance quality of life or sense of well-being. The body doesn't know what to do with food and fluids administered this way. Until fifty years ago, we never administered nutrition. The human body has not evolved to tolerate such feedings and thrive.

I try to have a thoughtful discussion, typically at the bedside, explaining to patients and families the real complications of these devices and interventions.

Family caregivers should anticipate and understand a number of other changes. Patients characteristically become cold to touch, especially the hands and the feet. Because there is a lowering of blood pressure, there is little merit to subjecting patients to multiple blood pressure readings. You can kindly ask the medical staff to stop taking the patient's blood pressure and pulse and respirations, especially if these patients are hooked up to monitors. Sometimes family members become fixated on the technology. It's not needed.

On the other hand, it is reasonable to keep on board interventions to enhance quality of life. The stool softener, the antidepressant, the sleeping pill do not dramatically change the natural history of the disease but certainly increase quality of life and the patient's sense of well-being. These decisions are fairly easy, but some decisions are not.

Let's suppose we're dealing with a midlife woman with far-advanced breast cancer who has shortness of breath, profound fatigue, and a hemoglobin of 6, which reflects the level of oxygen in the blood. A normal hemoglobin for most individuals is about 14. Without doubt, several pints of blood would make her feel far more comfortable, and there needs to be a thoughtful discussion with the medical team. Is this reasonable when the patient's survival might be limited to several weeks? I think so.

So as the dying process evolves, there needs to be a concerted effort to carefully review the patient's medications and ask which of these are mission-critical for quality of life and which are burdensome and do not enhance the remaining time that the patient has.

If patients are hallucinating or if they are not sleeping, there are well-established guidelines for using sedation medications. Delirium can be devastating for patients and families, and medications such as haloperidol are an important part of this order. There are also clear guidelines for medications to treat excessive secretions, as well as nausea and vomiting.

Many patients in the hospital are at risk for a deep venous thrombosis, or a blood clot, and typically receive anticoagulation drugs to prevent clots. But this is not appropriate for most dying patients.

I discuss pain management more deeply in a separate section, but suffice it to say, assessing and controlling pain must be first and foremost. The use of pain medications and related agents is very specific and quite clear: these agents address pain relief and quality of life and are not intended to hasten the patient's death. The goal of the medication is to relieve pain or discomfort or shortness of breath or hallucinations; the goal is not to hurry death.

Quality of Life and Death

I keep using the term *quality of life,* and here's why. In my work, that's my goal because quality of life can lead to quality of death. Studies funded by the National Institutes of Health have shown that palliative care can improve quality of life, even if the outcome is death. Patients at the end of life who were offered palliative care, usually pain management, reported fewer symptoms and less depression and anxiety than patients who received standard care.

Integrating palliative care into treatment plans is my mantra, and you will read more about that in upcoming pages.

An issue that arises occasionally is when the anguished family member asks, "Doc, I can't stand to see her suffer. Can't we do something to move this along?"

These sorts of inquiries require a thoughtful and face-to-face discussion between you, as caregiver, and the medical team to ensure that every measure will be taken to decrease discomfort, fully acknowledging that one of the anticipated and foreseeable side effects of morphine for pain might be respiratory depression. Understand that there's certainly no evidence that the careful and responsible use of pain medication hastens the patient's death.

We can easily envision a situation where a family member did not understand the concept of pain relief and the side effects of morphine, and therefore could interpret the patient's death as being accelerated or provoked by the morphine.

Continuing our earlier discussion, as the dying process progresses, we usually see a pale or bluish discoloration of the skin, and breathing becomes sporadic and erratic, punctuated by long pauses after which there is typically an audible gasp. A distressing phenomenon for family members is the death rattle, which consists of the gurgling sound typically caused by fluids pooling around the voice box. Almost never is this distressing to the patient, but, clearly, it can be disturbing to the family members.

A surprisingly common phenomenon that has been well described by patients is the sense of a trip or a journey through a tunnel, at the end of which there is typically an illuminated area like a beacon or a lighthouse or even just a ray of light. It's fascinating how common this phenomenon is. Many individuals acknowledge that deceased family members and friends, even pets, wait at the end of this tunnel, inviting the patient to "cross over" to the "other side"—or however they may define such an experience, if they can verbalize at all.

We've all heard and read about the out-of-body experience, and some individuals have even had a sense of sadness when they were called back from the other side in the midst of a successful resuscitation from a cardiac event. Some have described to me being called to the other side by a relative, typically a spouse, and there is a feeling of peace and light at the other end of the tunnel. These are universal experiences. I don't discount them.

Physically, the final end point in this journey is a cessation of breathing. There is no pulse, the heart stops, and death has occurred.

When I encounter family members sitting vigil at the bedsides of my patients in the hospital, I often see absolute exhaustion—the soul-shredding fatigue of family members as they keep that final vigil.

Although I'm not aware of hard data on this point, I have the distinct clinical impression that a high proportion of patients pass away after the family has left the room. What seems to be all too common is a bedside vigil of rotating family members to the point of exhaustion. They then leave the bedside for a cup of coffee or to attend to personal needs or take a cell phone call in the hallway, and then the patient passes away.

We can speculate as to the significance of this event. Again, I have no hard data, but it is a bedside observation also shared by other end-of-life medical colleagues.

Respect for Cultural Beliefs

Let me be crystal clear that there are profound cultural, societal, and historical nuances to the dying process that we must embrace and acknowledge. In some belief systems, life is precious, regardless of the quality of that life, and as long as there is the capacity to breathe and have a heartbeat, some cultures expect and demand that all life-sustaining measures will be continued. We in healthcare must be respectful of these divergent opinions.

It is simply not acceptable for some cultures to embark upon a palliative approach. Instead, there is a relentless attempt to explore every conceivable option, regardless of risks and regardless of relative futility. It is important for those of us on the care team to understand those cultures and be respectful of the patient's wishes and the desires of the family, even though we may not be in agreement with that approach. We ask that family members tell us about their special beliefs.

My first experience with cultural beliefs surrounding death occurred many years ago when there was an influx of boat people from Vietnam to Rochester, Minnesota. These refugees had endured unimaginable horror as they fled the communists, following the Vietnam War, some in tiny boats in the South China Sea. We welcomed them as warmly as possible, considering they were coming to the frigid tundra of Minnesota.

One gentleman was dying of advanced cancer and had state-of-the-art management. He was on a respirator and dialysis and multiple medications to maintain blood pressure, fight off infection, and keep him comfortable. He also had a catheter in his bladder to drain urine.

As death approached, the family became agitated, confused, and disoriented. They began wailing at his bedside. We asked one of the religious members of the Vietnamese community what was going on, and he shared with me that the way the patient was at death was the way he would spend eternity, and here he was, dying, with all these artificial interventions, in frozen Minnesota.

Once we knew this, we removed the devices so that the patient could be prepared for the way he would spend his afterlife. He was a barber, so he was fitted with scissors, a mirror, and a comb. To combat the frigid weather, he was provided with warm boots, a hat, gloves, and a coat. This looked bizarre to us, but the family was profoundly gratified that we acknowledged their belief system.

In some Native American cultures, once the patient has died, there are rituals of incense and candle burning. With the appropriate input of administration, these needs can often be met in a culturally sensitive manner, even in a hospital setting. We just need to know about them.

I can recall deaths among Asian patients, and there is a ritualized bathing of the deceased corpse. It's important that the eldest son appropriately attend to the body, and if these wishes are ignored, this can cause great anguish among survivors.

In the Roman Catholic community, for example, there is no ecclesiastical imperative to continue artificial hydration and nutrition when the burden exceeds the benefit or when there is no reasonable probability of reversing the process. Therefore, to withdraw artificial hydration and nutrition in this clinical setting has the support of church doctrine, which can be a tremendous source of peace and comfort to patients and family members.

In other belief systems, however, it is almost heresy to withdraw artificial hydration and nutrition. If there appears to be no reasonable probability of improvement, the input of the clergy for that belief system is absolutely crucial to assuage the guilt and the anguish of the patient and the family.

Let me circle back to the subject of this chapter and address the question of what death is, actually. In my world, and in the eyes of the American Medical Association and the American Bar Association, and in some form in all fifty states, a uniform determination includes wording about irreversible cessation of breathing and heartbeat and functions of the brain. With respirators now breathing for patients, that definition gets a little more imperfect.

If you are at the bedside when someone dies—when they have left us and passed on—you will know the answer to the question.

4

Don't We Have the Right to Die?

WE ARE A DEATH-DENYING CULTURE. JUST HOW FAR SHOULD medicine go in keeping someone alive—delaying death?

Now, we need to have some understanding of medical and historical precedent to understand where we are in contemporary American medicine on this moral, legal, and ethical question.

Some important landmark legal cases have provided a framework for difficult end-of-life decisions today. You may remember them.

In 1975, Karen Ann Quinlan of New Jersey lost consciousness after consuming alcohol and drugs at the age of twenty-one. She lapsed into a persistent vegetative state and was maintained on a ventilator and a feeding tube. The parents were consistent, public, and vocal in their belief that these interventions were not in line with their daughter's wishes. The doctors argued the other side.

The New Jersey Supreme Court ruled in favor of the patient and family in this right-to-die case, and the ventilator was removed. The parents allowed the feeding tube to continue, and the patient lived for eight additional years.

The next landmark case was Nancy Cruzan. In 1983, she was in a car accident at the age of twenty-six and was resuscitated at the scene. She had severe injuries and also lapsed into a persistent vegetative state. The parents contended their daughter did not want to be maintained in this condition on a feeding tube. The hospital refused to remove it.

The Missouri Supreme Court supported continuing the feeding tube, claiming that there was not clear and convincing evidence of the patient's wishes. However, information was collected from friends and family members to support the statement that the patient would not wish to be so maintained, and the feeding tube was removed. Nancy had told a friend earlier that year of her wishes. This case paved the way for attention to living wills and advance directives. (I discuss this in detail in chapters 21 and 22.)

The case of Terri Schiavo, which made headlines for fifteen years, underscores the importance of having someone designated to make healthcare decisions if you cannot make them for yourself and clearly compels everyone to spell out what they would do if they could not speak for themselves.

After a protracted and complex legal battle from 1990 to 2005, a Florida judge acted in accordance with the wishes of the patient and her husband, and the feeding tube was withdrawn. The patient died. An autopsy demonstrated extensive brain damage. The young woman's parents had been fighting to keep the feeding tube in place.

For these difficult ethical, legal, and moral issues, there is no algorithm or website, but there are some guiding principles that patients and family should consider:

- Who speaks for the patient, and is that patient being represented by the individual with their best interest in mind? A legal document (a living will or advance directive) is the definitive document. States have various hierarchies of decision-makers when patients no longer have what is called decisional capacity and when no advance directive has been completed. These "default surrogates" may be ranked as related by blood, marriage, or adoption, and include spouse, child, and parent (some allow partner or chosen adult, same-sex partner, domestic partner, interested person, friend). You can see how things get sticky quickly. And then imagine a scenario where a patient is from one state and being treated in another state with different hierarchies of decision-makers.

- There needs to be a compassionate and respectful family conference at some point with the medical care team, where the key stakeholders—family members—can express their concerns and enlist the input of the patient if that's feasible. Otherwise, the patient's representative can act on their behalf.

- You should expect your care team to clearly summarize your family conferences in the patient's record and write down exactly what was discussed and who said it, since during times of stress and fatigue there is often selective amnesia, which can lead to significant misunderstandings among family members. I've seen it and often felt I should have been wearing a referee's whistle.

Dying on Your Own Terms

We need to recognize the right of self-determination. Elizabeth Bouvia was a woman living in a nursing home, with severe cerebral palsy and a nasal gastric feeding tube and a dreadful pain situation. The patient understood that she was being sustained by the artificial hydration and nutrition through the tube and requested that the court order her caregivers to remove the tube. She wanted to die by starving herself to death.

In the mid-1980s, Bouvia's was a landmark case in the right-to-die movement. A higher court eventually agreed with her request, and this was consistent with the legal precedent of the patient's right "to be left alone." She actually survived and was still alive in 2008.

So even though a specific treatment or intervention may be curative, if the patient refuses that intervention and if the patient is aware of the consequences, it is the patient's right to refuse that treatment or that technology.

We on the medical team—and the family members too—need to honor and support this right.

5

Why Does a Person's Life Story Matter at the End of Life?

EVERYONE HAS A STORY. EVERYONE HAS A HISTORY. FOR example, I met a disabled elderly gentleman in the intensive care unit. He had cancer. No one bothered to find out about his profession. When I asked what he did, his family shared with me that he was the inventor of the wheeled knife used to cut pizza. Rather than focus on the grim reality of his diagnosis and the outcome we all knew was ahead, I talked with him and his family about cutting pizza.

For more than forty years, I have had the privilege of meeting incredible people like this and hearing their stories. They are my patients. I am their doctor. But not their first doctor. You see, when patients come to Mayo Clinic, the doctor they see may be their second opinion or their tenth, more likely their third or fourth. They are desperate for answers, and they are often gravely ill.

The businessman sitting next to you on the airplane. The clerk at the grocery store. The postal carrier. The business owner. The minister. A farmer. A professor. A nurse. A computer programmer. A chef. A roofer. A truck driver. A teacher. A mom or dad. A hairdresser. A grandma or grandpa. The inventor of the pizza cutter. These are my patients. In daily life, they are faceless people we may never know. But in the exam room, I come to know them personally.

When we physicians and healthcare providers interact with a patient, that patient brings to the examination room an illness—perhaps cancer or heart disease or a psychiatric problem—and that illness is wrapped in an envelope reflecting the patient's past experiences, history, and life's journey.

I can't speak for my medical colleagues, but I need to know something about that individual—their life's work, their family situation, their understanding of their medical problems, their fears, and their expectations. I always ask about their educational background and their livelihood, along with some context of where they live and who they are as people. I even know the name of their dog. In that way, I never treat a patient as a number or a file or a disease. I am treating a fellow human being who has a name and a history and a family.

By the same token, we physicians bring to the bedside our own experiences. So let me share with you some of my background and provide the context of how my journey as a cancer doctor and end-of-life specialist has unfolded.

Family histories often become blurred and obscured by time and memories. But this is mine. In the early 1900s, a refugee ship left the gritty, gray seaport of Hamburg, Germany, with about 3,000 immigrants hoping to seek a better life. One of those immigrants was a ten- or twelve-year-old boy who spoke not a word of English and whose parents made the ultimate sacrifice of scraping together a sum of money to put him on that ship for a better life.

We do not know the specifics of his early years, but, like most young men at that time in history, he was destined to be conscripted into the German army and would have faced a brutal existence as life unfolded at that time in Eastern Europe. We know from family records that his name was Harry Stiles Stahl, and through some circumstances, he wound up in Bucks County, Pennsylvania, just north of Philadelphia. But now for the rest of the fascinating story.

Local legends indicated that Harry, as a young man, was fearless around horses and was small in stature. As he reached his teenage years, he was no more than about 5 feet, 5 inches tall, and topped out at about 120 pounds. He developed a local reputation for training and racing horses and was encouraged by his patrons to have enough courage to leave Pennsylvania and head for the big time in New York and New Jersey.

A faded photograph from the *Newark Ledger* showed the young, talented horseman at Head's Stable. He then developed a successful career as a prominent jockey on the East Coast. He was an entrepreneur, a street-smart and savvy businessman, and was one of the first race riders to hire a valet who acted as his agent and manager and coordinated his silks, his boots, and his racing tack. Harry was my grandfather.

I lived with him until his death in the early 1950s, and I vividly recall living a privileged life. He had a magnificent oceanfront estate in Deal, New Jersey, about one hour south of New York City, where he lived the life of a rock star. But then, the wheels came off, and his career came to a crushing halt because, like many young men with lots of talent but not a lot of common sense, his weight started to balloon. He started to drink on a regular basis and became an abusive alcoholic. He spent his remaining years working at a refinery in a steel mill, and it was not a pretty picture.

The message I got very clearly as a young boy was that if our physical health deteriorates, we lose our ability to make a living, and the outcome will not be appealing. That's exactly what happened to my grandfather.

Another immigrant left Europe at about the same time. The Irish peasant during the early part of the 1900s was one of the most impoverished and marginalized and downtrodden reflections of humanity in the world. It's difficult for us to contemplate what life was like during Irish history. We all vaguely remember that the great famine took place in the middle part of the 1800s, and although the numbers are somewhat imprecise, several million Irish starved to death.

My grandmother was age eleven when, one bitterly cold and dreary Irish night, her parents awakened her and gave her a choice: in the morning a horse-drawn wagon would be at the end of the lane, headed to Cove, the harbor of Cork, where a ship would be leaving for America. My grandmother was clearly told that if she remained in Ireland, she would undoubtedly die from consumption, which was another name for tuberculosis, or she would starve to death, or she would die under the oppression of the British boot.

By grace or a miracle or some higher power, my grandmother made that decision to leave her family, with the full understanding and recognition that she would never return to Ireland and would never again see her family.

I was raised by my grandmother, that girl who left Ireland at age eleven, all alone. Everything she owned in this world was in a pillowcase that she carried onto the ship. She spent almost a month at sea, crossing the North Atlantic in the middle of winter. She never saw the light of day, since she was below decks with other steerage passengers in the hull of the ship. The death rate of the Irish crossing the Atlantic at that time in history was about 30 percent. In other words, a third never even made it to America, having died from dysentery, tuberculosis, and other infectious diseases during the crossing.

She was dumped on Ellis Island like a piece of luggage, along with millions of other immigrants, and spoke not one word of English. She only spoke Irish (Gaelic). She shared with me that her first job was as a domestic for a prominent New York City family.

One day, she was given a watermelon to prepare. In Ireland everything was boiled. My grandmother had never seen a watermelon, so this Irish waif dropped the green missile into a vat of boiling water. You don't have to be a physicist to anticipate what happened. The explosion sounded like a train going through the living room, and the seeds were embedded in the ceilings, the upholstery, and throughout the kitchen.

My grandmother was terrified that she would be put out on the street, and you can imagine what a nightmare this was for a young immigrant who didn't speak English. It is these sorts of stories and experiences that make us who we are today.

Like my grandfather, she was street-smart and savvy; she knew how to work the system, and she survived. What I learned from these two characters was self-reliance.

A fascinating and sometimes ignored measure of the end-of-life situation is to ask our loved ones about their life story. Once that person passes away, that rich tapestry of history, heritage, and tradition will evaporate. With smartphones and video making it so easy to capture words and images, these bedside chats may reveal details long hidden away in memories.

For better or for worse, we inherit, at least to some extent, the values and the hopes and the disappointments of our parents. My mother—the product of these two stalwarts—was a wonderful woman who had a caring and compassionate philosophy to those less fortunate, but she struggled mightily with alcoholism. As a young boy, her struggle gave me some insight that alcoholism was not a choice; it was an illness, much like diabetes or high blood pressure, and required professional intervention, which was hardly available at that time in history.

My biological father also struggled with alcoholism and never achieved a consistent sobriety. But in his own way, he was a savant. By that I mean he had a very narrow and deep area of expertise and became fanatical and maniacal about analyzing past performances of racehorses. He had elaborate notebooks filled with every nuance and subtlety of a horse's performance and made a successful living at the racetracks, primarily on the East Coast. And for a time, his handicapping and predictive skills were so uncanny that he represented jockeys to trainers. And for that he received a handsome cut of what the jockey made.

So how did these experiences impact upon me as a health-care provider? Money, prestige, bank accounts, and professional acknowledgments all become irrelevant and fade into the background if our health goes south. I also learned that we need to take care of ourselves physically, spiritually, and emotionally, and we cannot expect to hit the lottery or hope that a hot horse will provide the big payoff to eliminate the mortgage or other financial obligations.

My parents were divorced when I was about eight. Just think for a moment what it must have been like for a single, divorced, Roman Catholic woman with a young child in the New York/ New Jersey area in the 1950s. This phenomenon has defined the American culture of today, but this was a dreadful indictment of one's morality back in the 1950s. This was simply unacceptable, and it made my mother a tough, defiant, and resilient individual. Perhaps I inherited some of her characteristics.

My mother's second husband, Willie, whose story I have already shared, owned bars and liquor stores outside of New York City. I tell audiences that I have learned more from my days in those bars than from any sociology or psychology course I ever took. I spent many hours in these "temples of sin" and have memories of individuals who talked about great skills and great talents but complained that they never achieved greatness or stardom because of bad luck. The recurring theme was about *what could have been, but the manager shafted me or my wife would never support me; I was on my way to Carnegie Hall or I could have been president of Harvard,* but...and there was always a *but.*

So what I heard and what I vividly remember were excuses, and as I reflect on those individuals, they never really took responsibility for their own personal miseries. I wasn't the most insightful little boy, but I still have memories of people who always blamed somebody else for their misfortunes, and I hope that has given me some insight, both personally and professionally, that we need to have a firm hand on the wheel of our own lives and cannot blame others for the way things turn out—although I often hear these themes from dying patients at the bedside.

Whether our parents were butchers, bakers, or candlestick makers, we cannot escape their influence upon us, both for better and for worse. For me, one of the most powerful influences in my early years was life at the tracks. Our world involved the racetracks of Miami, namely Hialeah, Calder, Tropical, and Gulfstream; the spring racing meets at Pimlico in Maryland; and then the summer and fall season in New Jersey, including Garden State, Monmouth Park, Atlantic City, and then the races in New York, including Belmont, Aqueduct, and Saratoga.

Our lives revolved around which track was open and finding the next hot horse. Most of the focus was in New Jersey, since this was where we spent most of our time. The patrons of my stepfather's bar were a bizarre collection of the human gene pool: grooms, hot walkers, jockeys, valets, agents, exercise riders, kitchen staff, and the other nameless faces who kept the track operating.

In a bizarre world like that, as a little boy it is almost impossible to sort out what's normal versus what's abnormal versus what's absolutely bizarre and wacko. I can recall many a holiday season watching the *Lawrence Welk Show,* or related activities with Santa Claus and presents and a Christmas tree, and wondering if that was reality or if reality was being surrounded by people who had fallen off the wagon and whose lives were a complete mess.

But the grace or the gift that I was somehow given was to understand that there was a better way. There was another life, and that key to the kingdom clearly rested with athletic and academic performance.

Being an only child and living in my grandmother's rooming house, again with some bizarre people, made me understand that this was not a life path I wished to take. I was blessed in being orthopedically sound and had the gift to run distance races. I had considerable visibility and success as a distance runner in New Jersey high schools and was able to have some success throughout college and medical school, but I clearly understood one fact: athletic greatness is a fading ember. It is a skill set that is quickly evaporated by age and injury, and I somehow knew deep in my soul that the ticket out of this curious world was through academic achievement.

I created a fanatical study habit, and I can vividly recall my time in college, basically sitting almost motionless for six hours studying difficult subjects like physics, math, and organic chemistry. Failure was absolutely not an option, and I knew that with focus on and penetration of the subject, I could achieve a level of mastery.

The college years were incredibly difficult because, at LaSalle College in Philadelphia, most of the premed students had come from the premier, highly selective high schools throughout the Philadelphia area. They had extensive backgrounds in math and science and biology, and I felt ill prepared to compete with them, based upon my education at a small Catholic school outside of New York City. But I somehow knew that with intense focus and dedication I could shift the odds in my favor, and that is indeed what happened.

So what I learned at the track is that there is no such thing as luck. We make our luck. For me, life at the track and in rooming houses and bus depots brought the grimness of life into short reality. Few made it to the top of the gene pool in that environment, while others languished in obscurity and a fog of alcoholism. That was not a life I chose, and I tried to get far from it, yet I remembered the lessons I had learned about compassion and caring.

Now, as a medical professional, I have been present at the bedside for many patients—each with a story. What I have learned from this is that who you are shapes your legacy at the end of your life. We all want to look back with no regrets.

6

What Do We Do When the Doctor Delivers Bad News?

MEDICINE, OBVIOUSLY, IS BOTH AN ART AND A SCIENCE. THE competent clinician—whether an MD or a DO or an RN or a midlevel provider—must master certain facts and a body of knowledge. But some knowledge is not taught to us in medical school. Or not practiced well, because breaking bad news to families or delivering devastating news to patients is a lot more art than science. These conversations contain that underlying current of the shattering news that life will end imminently.

Until recently, most healthcare providers had absolutely no background in how to compassionately and effectively break bad news. If you've ever been on the receiving end of a dire phone call about a loved one or a scary diagnosis in the exam room, you can play that movie over and over in your head because it's burned into your memory.

Having been touched by tens of thousands of encounters with the terminally ill, I have developed some strategies that help me deliver bad news with compassion. In my line of work, such responsibilities weigh heavily on me, and I approach the task with great solemnity. Let me share with you how I handle this difficult situation. I acknowledge that you may not be on the receiving end of similar compassion in discussing grave health situations. But you and your loved ones deserve to be.

In medical literature, the term SPIKES has been extensively reviewed. These letters refer to

S the *setting* for the breaking of bad news;
P the patient's *perception* of the conversation;
I obtaining the patient's *invitation* (how much information the patient actually wants);
K the patient's *knowledge* base;
E awareness of the patient's *emotions* (which includes the medical team's responding with empathy); and
S the *summary* of these elements.

Let's explore the elements of SPIKES one by one.

Setting

It's important that the encounter be shared with patient and family in a safe, secure environment free from distractions. The clinician who answers a pager or accesses a tablet or a cell phone erodes the energy and the karma of the interchange. If you are on the receiving end of such dire conversations, it is appropriate for you to say, "Let's move this conversation to a private room" or "Doctor, could we close the door for some privacy while we discuss this?" You can reasonably even say this: "I am not really at peace with this conversation. Is there someone else I can speak to who can provide another perspective on the problem?"

Perception

It's important for your medical team to understand your perception of the problem. I often ask this: "Please share with me what your doctors have told you." That way, I show that I want and need to know where the patient and family are in terms of understanding the medical situation. Then, together, we can start the care conversation wherever you are in your own understanding.

Instead, you might typically be asked, "What do you know about your condition?" This clearly puts the burden on the patient and family. Ask questions of your care team even if you think you may sound uninformed. You are swimming in an entirely new ocean of medical terms and diagnoses. You deserve to understand.

Invitation

Next, we need to discern how much information the patient actually wants. In some cultures, all decisions are referred to a family member, and that's okay, but in many Westernized communities, patients want all the facts and figures to help them make a decision.

Now, these sorts of discussions apply to the typical American family, whatever that means to most of us. However, the care team must understand the cultural, geographic, and historical context of the patient. For example, in some cultures, it is simply not acceptable and, in fact, almost forbidden to share a diagnosis of "cancer" with the patient. This can be viewed as punishment from a higher power, with devastating implications for the patient and the family.

If we caregivers are not familiar with your culture, we need to inform ourselves and learn from the responsible family member how this issue should be addressed. We appreciate when a family member explains these nuances in advance. In some cultures, it is perfectly acceptable to say there is a spot or a shadow on the X-ray, and then respectfully sidestep the specific term of *cancer*.

I know that among Native American and some Asian patients, many would not want to know a specific prognosis, and the care team must be sensitive to that cultural nuance. When language is a barrier, it is not satisfactory in most circumstances for a family member to act as the interpreter. Ideally, a certified language consultant should be brought to the bedside or to the examination room so that there is a clear understanding of the medical issues. Hospitals are required to provide interpreters in a patient's native language. You must ask for such services if required or if the provider doesn't immediately recognize the need.

Knowledge

I ask the patient, "What do you understand about the current situation?" Their understanding may be completely mistaken, whether too optimistic or simply in error in terms of dealing with the reality of their illness. Let me explain.

William had advanced cancer of the colon, which was resected (the diseased portion removed), but eighteen lymph nodes adjacent to the cancer contained malignant cells, and a nodule in the liver, which harbored cancer, was taken out. When I asked him what he understood about his situation, he replied, "Well, everything was removed. Nothing was left behind, so I am in pretty good shape."

He understood that the cancer was removed from the colon, but any reasonable person could understand the incredibly high probability of recurrence because of the cancer in the liver and in eighteen lymph nodes. This knowledge prompted a very different type of discussion involving probably bad news.

Emotions

I cannot overemphasize the importance of empathy. This is the gift of honoring the patient's emotions, trying to understand where that patient is and what it would feel like to walk a mile in their shoes. Patients have shared with me that we, as healthcare providers, cannot possibly empathize with patients in the truest sense, but we certainly can share several phrases of value. I often say, "I cannot imagine how difficult this is for you." When appropriate, I may also say something like this: "Just look at where you have come from in the past couple of weeks. You were fit and healthy, but then you suddenly became fatigued and developed a lump in your neck, and now, here we are, talking about advanced cancer."

One patient told me that a cancer doctor said, "There's nothing more we can do for you." After handing the patient a tissue, the doctor exited the exam room, saying only, "Stay in here as long as you need." Again, I cannot account for the seemingly uncaring actions of medical colleagues. There is no excuse. This was completely insensitive. Do not let the physician leave with such a flippant comment. There are always options and alternatives. Say this: "Guide me. Don't abandon me." These situations often lead to patients futilely seeking second and third opinions, either in the same institution or in a different city or medical center.

Summary:

It's also important to end with a crisp summary to the patient and family. Done well, the doctor might end the conversation with something like this: "Okay, let me now step back, take a 30,000-foot view, and relay exactly where we are. Are there any questions that I did not ask? Is there anything else?"

Have your questions in mind. Ask them. Take notes. Now is the time. And you may appropriately respond, "What questions have we not asked that we should ask?"

I often ask patients this question: "What are you most concerned about?" The answer may surprise the medical care team and the family because what the family and physicians are concerned about may be quite different from the patient's concerns. I often find patients more concerned about taking care of a surviving spouse or a pet at home than about their own well-being.

If all goes well during these difficult situations when bad news is delivered and discussed, you will understand what's going on. Patients and caregivers need to feel validated and acknowledged, not adrift in a medical sea without a flotation device.

7

"Doc, How Long Do I Have to Live?"

THE UNSPOKEN QUESTION FOR MANY OF MY PATIENTS AND THEIR families toward the end of life goes something like this: "Okay, Doc, how long do I have?" This is an emotionally charged issue that I handle with tact and diplomacy.

But let me explain how the answer to this question becomes very complicated and why your care team cannot predict, nor should they.

For most conditions, such as heart disease, kidney failure, and cancer, there are some reasonably predictable observations and tests and scans that help predict how long a patient will live. However, these are ballpark figures, are rarely precise, and really cannot give a specific answer because each patient is different, and many factors affect survival.

Studies show, for example, that there is a downturn in deaths among Jewish gentlemen at the time of the High Holy Days in autumn, and then, following the holy days, there is an upward spike in deaths. So what does this mean? It means that some individuals in a certain belief system become energized, have a focus to survive, and look forward to the religious ceremony and the gathering of family and friends. Perhaps there's a surge of cortisone or other types of hormones that energize the patients temporarily, and then they pass away.

We have often heard about the experience of a patient just hanging on until there is that visit from the prodigal son or the estranged daughter. The patient is then at peace and dies. I've seen this over and over in clinical settings. But let me get more specific.

It is vitally important that patients and families have some understanding of prognosis. The prognosis is the expected outcome or forecast about the condition.

When patients have an unreasonably optimistic estimate of survival, they generally favor more aggressive, potentially dangerous, and invasive interventions, some studies show. For example, I am reminded of a gentleman in his early forties who had a viral infection of his heart that developed into a condition called cardiomyopathy. This simply meant that the pumping chambers of the heart became weakened and flabby, and the patient was short of breath and had swelling of the legs and was miserable.

Yet he had an unrealistic estimate of his survival and was willing to undergo all sorts of experimental drug treatments to bolster the pumping of the heart. He did not do well, and his remaining time was not quality filled.

On the other hand, his family shared with his healthcare team that if he had known how grave the prognosis was and how limited his survival time, he would not have been willing to undergo these incredibly painful and unsuccessful interventions.

So patients and families need to be appropriately assertive in trying to get some ballpark figure for the patient's survival. If you watch many daytime soap operas and TV medical shows, the doctors always give the patient "six months." But this is unrealistic. There is another way of reframing prognosis that I have personally found helpful. Let me explain.

Let's suppose a patient has a diagnosis of advanced lung cancer and, because of a variety of factors, his prognosis is estimated to be approximately six to eight months. These estimates are just that: estimates. They are based on how other patients have done in the same disease state.

A technique that I have found helpful is to reframe prognosis in terms of events, holidays, and celebrations. For example, if the patient had a prognosis of six months in January and he was an avid fisherman, I might say that by the time the fishing opener came around—mid-May in Minnesota—we should be prepared for some major setbacks. Another way of reframing this would be to say that by the time we get near Memorial Day, we really should be prepared for some major setbacks.

This technique works with families who, instead of counting days and weeks and months, have an undefined target, such as "holiday time" or "fall" or "when the weather starts to warm up." When a patient and family put the prognosis into perspective this way, instead of counting days on the calendar, plans can be made without pressure and presumption. Obviously, if the average survival time is six months, many people live much longer; of course, it also means that others do not live that long.

There is another reason why this prognosis discussion is so important. I can recall a painful circumstance where a patient had far-advanced cancer of the liver. The patient had a condition called ascites, meaning that the abdominal cavity was filled with fluid. The patient's arms and legs were wasted, almost like sticks, and the patient was deeply jaundiced with almost a greenish discoloration. The prognosis was obviously very serious, and I outlined as best I could, based on the information that we had, that the prognosis, at best, was perhaps a short number of months. The patient and family seemed satisfied with that discussion and left for home.

Several weeks later, I received a thoughtful letter from the family that the patient had died approximately three weeks after our consultation. I felt badly about this situation, since I had overestimated the patient's prognosis. I called the family and expressed my condolences and my regrets, and the family was grateful for the information and the care that the patient had received.

Now, why is this a big deal? Well, if patients and families recognize that the prognosis is short, that the quality of life may well deteriorate, there are then opportunities to close chapters. To make amends, to reach out with that olive branch, seeking reconciliation for past indiscretions or unfortunate circumstances.

To make time to close doors, open new doors, forgive and be forgiven, it's reasonable for patients and family to question the healthcare team about length of survival. But, rather than asking for a specific number, which can be misleadingly unrealistic, simply ask whether or not the patient might be here for the holiday season or for Mother's Day or for the next Super Bowl. This gives patients and families a target—a span of time during which to do the important work of healing the lesions of the soul.

Another dimension of the prognosis discussion is for us on the medical side to simply ask the patient this: *Why is this question important to you at this time in your illness?* The person's response can offer a rich dialogue of unspoken concerns that need to be addressed and reconciled as their physical condition deteriorates.

For some conditions, such as advanced cancer, it is somewhat easier and more accurate to estimate prognosis the sicker the patient becomes. But for other conditions, such as heart disease and emphysema/chronic obstructive pulmonary disease (COPD), patients often bounce back from a hospitalization but often do not return to their previous baseline of functioning. For any given hospital stay, it is really not possible to accurately estimate prognosis.

Another important dimension of this issue is to caution you about accessing websites that offer tools to estimate prognosis. This exercise can be terrifying for patients and typically reflects broad populations of individuals who have varying degrees of fitness. For example, a thirty-year-old patient with advanced lung cancer generally has a far better prognosis than a seventy-year-old patient with advanced lung cancer, yet these patients may be lumped together in a broad statistical review of survival.

I never discourage patients and families from seeking information, but I do offer that important warning that the internet provides too broad a view of an issue, and the numbers can be profoundly misleading.

The Problem with Optimism

A fascinating article in the *New York Times* of May 2013 addressed the issue of cancer optimism. This is a complex issue, but to demystify it, please read on.

When physicians and other medical professionals are unreasonably optimistic and hopeful for a positive result from an intervention whether it is surgery, an artificial heart, or some experimental medicine, patients are more prone to go down that road.

By nature, we caregivers overestimate prognosis. We often overestimate the benefit of treatment, and patients trust us. In their minds and in the minds of the family, the risks are outweighed by the potential benefits, but that's not necessarily the case.

I have a vivid memory of a courageous fifty-six-year-old homemaker from North Carolina. Ella was a prominent businesswoman in her community and engaged in her medical care. She had a type of cancer common among smokers called small cell cancer or oat cell cancer. The cancer had spread to some lymph nodes behind the breastbone in an area called the mediastinum, and it was certainly reasonable to proceed with chemotherapy and radiation, which was the gold standard for management.

She did well and the scans showed a dramatic shrinkage of the cancer although there was the hint of some residual disease.

These are unsettling situations for which there is no hard and fast recommendation. The tendency, the trend is to recommend additional cycles of what are called consolidative chemotherapy. In other words, this is a type of treatment involving toxic intravenous drugs designed to "mop up" any cancer cells that were not killed by the original treatment.

Ella had lost some weight. Her activity level was marginal, and her appetite was not ideal. Equally important, her husband had been in an automobile accident, so he was not available to her. He had been her rock, her support, during this difficult time.

With some uneasiness on our part, but encouragement from Ella who wanted to get better to help her husband, the backup chemotherapy was started and the situation did not go well. She developed low blood counts, as often happens. Her immune system could not bounce back, and she had multiple hospital admissions for bloodstream infections, one of which caused an erosion of a heart valve requiring emergency surgery.

So here we have the typical situation where the patient's perception of the recommendation was far more positive and far more optimistic than was warranted. This is a delicate line that we walk with our patients. This is a tightrope. On one hand, you may be offered legitimate treatment options, but many times we send that message in an envelope of optimism, which can often cause some serious complications and decreased quality of life as it did in this patient.

So how do we as doctor and patient (and patient's family) navigate through these profound ethical and professional dilemmas? I believe that the most reasonable approach is to try to be factual. I meet my patients where they are in terms of terminology and vocabulary and clearly bring to the table other stakeholders such as members of the patient's family. That's why I need to know who my patients are. I want to know their story.

We often share numbers and percentages and probabilities with our patients, but I find that approach unsettling. A typical comment is that the risk of the treatment, whether it is surgical or medical, is 1 percent. Well, what patients do not understand— if they happen to be in that 1 percent—is that the outcome is hardly ideal.

Another dimension of the prognosis discussion is often not clearly stated. Multiple studies in the medical journals clearly document that we healthcare providers dramatically *overestimate* prognosis.

The overly optimistic prognosis becomes more apparent the closer the relationship between the physician and the patient. That lifelong relationship is especially evident in primary care and internal medicine because the physician has probably been treating the patient for many years. Their relationship distorts the reality of the medical problem. In general, the more intense and intimate that professional relationship is, the more optimistic the provider can be.

At a recent palliative medicine board review course in Louisville, I was struck by one of the presenters who made the comment that we in oncology overestimate prognosis by a factor of two or three. So if the physician estimates that the prognosis is six weeks of survival, in fact, the survival may only be two to three weeks.

The other issue with unreasonable optimism is that patients sometimes do not do the heavy lifting of resolving conflicts because they don't consider how grave their situation is.

I can recall some painful discussions with family members around the bedside as the patient lapsed into a coma and was deteriorating from a combination of advanced cancer, multiple internal medical conditions such as heart and kidney disease compounded by the complications of treatment. Families have occasionally told me that they would have had those hard conversations sooner had they realized how ill the patient was and how rapidly the patient would be deteriorating.

"What Would You Do, Doc?"

Another dimension of this issue is a question I commonly hear, and it goes something like this: "Okay, Doc, you've given me a lot of information and a lot of options, and I thank you for that, but at the end of the day, if it was your father, what would you do?" "If you were me, what would you do?"

I try to explain to patients and families that we cannot trade places. I obviously have insight and experience that gives me a different perspective on the situation, but that does not put me directly in the shoes of that patient or their family. In addition, these sorts of questions do not take into account that we each have a personal moral philosophy of how far to go in sustaining our lives.

Not many of my colleagues would say this, but I will. Although I have not been faced with some of these life-altering and life-consuming crises, my own belief at this quiet moment on a rainy Thursday morning as I write this is that I do not believe I would follow the aggressive road that many patients follow. I have seen the devastation to family members. I have seen firsthand the suffering not only of the patient but also of the family and of the community trying to support the patient and the family in the face of overwhelmingly negative odds. Let me give you a specific example.

One of our patients was a gentleman from rural Georgia whose congestive heart failure persisted despite every reasonable medication. He was a candidate for a left ventricular assist device from a cardiac perspective. In other words, his overall medical condition was such that this mechanical intervention would be reasonable. However—

He lived in a very small community with no practical access to medical care. His lifelong partner was a wonderfully supportive person but was not medically or technically sophisticated. She obviously wanted to do the right thing but was completely overwhelmed with the responsibility of managing the well-recognized complications of this device. The patient did undergo surgery, and it was successful, but his course at home was punctuated by multiple complications, which his partner was unable to handle.

So an important aspect of the decision for the patient is to recognize that they indeed are the focus of the treatment, but there is a ripple effect. There is a spinoff that cannot be ignored—namely, the impact of that patient's decision on the entire family. In other words, gather all the information from the medical team in order to make an informed choice, always understanding that in complex end-of-life situations there will be ramifications and consequences.

8
May I Share My Story about Palliative Care?

I'M A BOARD-CERTIFIED MEDICAL ONCOLOGIST, ONE OF THE first formally trained cancer specialists in the early 1970s. Prior to that, many physicians dabbled in cancer treatment but did not have any formal training. I received my board certification in 1977.

Jump ahead forty years. We are now facing a real cancer crisis in this country. At a time when there are about a third as many cancer specialists as we had even a decade ago, we have a tsunami of cancer patients as a result of the aging of the American population, since cancer is often a disease of aging.

Equally important, depending upon the source, about half of medical oncologists within the next several years will either quit this specialty or decrease their hours because of stress or burnout.

My stepfather, Willie, whose story I shared earlier, had very little symptom management for his pain and shortness of breath as he lay dying. This was the early 1990s. I'm not being critical. This was simply the state of the art of end-of-life management then. I made a commitment to myself that there must be a better way to do this.

A real epiphany occurred to me when I was seeing patients with far-advanced head and neck cancers. These patients typically receive aggressive radiation therapy Monday through Friday, over a five- to six-week period, and that's associated with difficult side effects of sores in the mouth, fatigue, and weight loss. The chemotherapy is often combined with radiation, and while this can be curative in a minority of patients, the treatment can accelerate their suffering.

Few discussions took place in doctors' lounges, in hospital hallways, or even at professional meetings about alleviating these distressing side effects and end-of-life suffering. I felt profound moral distress when I considered the poor quality of life of those patients.

At about the same time, quite by serendipity, I attended a meeting of hospice colleagues. These were primarily nurses, and I was introduced to some basic, scientifically sound methods for increasing quality of life, such as the use of steroids (also called prednisone or dexamethasone). Now, these were not new medicines, but we in oncology rarely used them.

To enhance the quality of life of these suffering patients, I started to use prednisone and was astonished at how much better they felt. They were also better able to tolerate treatment. This was my first eye-opener that we could do better by using relatively simple measures.

At that time, there was nearly no formal training in what became known as palliative medicine. It was primarily a mom-and-pop operation. However, in 1997 the palliative-medicine certifying examination was offered for the first time. I remember this day vividly. The examination was being offered at the University of Minnesota, on a bitterly cold morning, at a venue about a hundred miles from my home in Rochester, Minnesota.

As I drove to the test site, I became enveloped in a blinding snowstorm with frozen roads and virtually no visibility. As I made my way up the highway, I asked myself, *Am I completely nuts? This is absolute insanity to push on to simply take an exam.* However, the weather cleared. I did take the exam, and I passed. I had no idea the avenues and the doors and the roads that exam would open up.

So where does palliative medicine fit into the big picture at the end of life?

Most of us are familiar with the concept of the internist or internal-medicine physician. Under that generic umbrella are a number of subspecialists, such as the cardiologist (heart specialist), the nephrologist (kidney specialist), and the pulmonologist (lung specialist). And so on. And now palliative medicine is one of these recognized subspecialties.

The examination was offered in 2005, and I passed it; it was offered again in 2012, and I passed it. I really viewed these credentials with a tremendous sense of achievement, as well as being acknowledged as a Fellow of the American Academy of Hospice and Palliative Medicine.

Now, why is this such a big deal? The evolution of this specialty is an enormous deal because of the complexity and the aging of the baby boomers, as well as the sweeping changes in our social fabric.

We in southeast Minnesota have some of the most courageous and remarkable patients on the planet. Typically, an elderly patient was admitted to the hospital and had an acute crisis averted through surgery or medications, such as the management of a heart attack, pneumonia, or stroke. Once upon a time, that patient returned to their environment, which was most likely a small community or a farm, and the patient was surrounded by his or her loving family and was cared for.

Today, families are scattered. The cohesion that was once the hallmark of the agrarian society is eroding, and now we are confronted with the blended family, the split family, stepchildren, second wives, third husbands, life partners, pets, and all kinds of assorted relationships that profoundly complicate the problem of who will care for Grandpa when the Mayo Clinic sends him home to recover or live out his life comfortably.

Here is another issue. Once upon a time, every patient had a primary care provider like Dr. Marcus Welby. Dr. Welby was a TV doctor played by the venerable Robert Young. Welby had a charming bedside manner, made house calls, knew all his patients, and cured practically everything. The show ran from 1969 to 1976 and dominated Tuesday-night network TV before cable. *Marcus Welby, M.D.* was among the first of the blockbuster doctor shows.

I recall many circumstances during my early clinical years when we would ask that patient's Dr. Welby to come to the bedside to help with difficult decision-making. Today, this is hardly the case. Many patients do not have a primary care provider. They do not have a family practice physician or family doc, and they are overwhelmed by an armada of highly technical, specifically trained subspecialists who take a narrow view of the patient and may not understand the patient's psychosocial setting.

So a role for the palliative care community is to act as the interpreter, the translator, the quarterback—the one who brings to the patient and the family a reasonable interpretation in addressing the pros, cons, risks, and benefits of a bewildering number of highly technical and sometimes dangerous treatments. In short, the one who treats the whole person, not just the disease.

Here's an example: Incredible advances have been made in the management of heart disease. A number of decades ago, patients often died of an electrical event where there was a short-circuiting of the heart. The rhythm was erratic and chaotic, and the patients died. This was the typical patient who "dropped dead" or died in their sleep.

However, with advances in technology, such as implantable defibrillators, many of these patients are being saved from heart events that used to kill them and now, unfortunately, are dying from pump failure or congestive heart failure. This means that the pumping capacity of the heart is dramatically compromised. Patients retain fluid in their lungs, liver, and legs and are profoundly fatigued. They have general body pain, are short of breath, and have a dreadful quality of life. In some circumstances, these patients are candidates for a mechanical heart, also called a left ventricular assist device.

These lifesaving interventions are not without some risks, as mentioned. We in the palliative care community visit with these patients up front before surgery is done to explain, in conjunction with the surgeon and the cardiologist, the implications of this technology. If things do not go well, as sometimes happens, we can step up to the plate. The patients know us, and we can address symptoms and concerns as complications ensue.

But who is truly listening? Many patients and families are understandably "deaf" and do not remember or do not recall the complications of these procedures. We are then faced with the painful situation of how to handle these devices when they are no longer working and the patient is miserable from our technology.

Are these patients at the end of life? Most assuredly. Palliative care, which has been monitoring this patient all along, is there to provide symptom relief as medical events unfold. The cornerstone of the palliative care consultation is to address these distressing symptoms that include but are not limited to shortness of breath, difficulty in swallowing, weight loss and not eating, fatigue, nausea and vomiting, constipation, and delirium.

The palliative medicine consultant is specifically trained to drill into the nuances and the subtleties of management, and you can expect a palliative consult to take a careful, targeted history and physical examination and address in a meaningful manner techniques to help with these complaints and concerns.

As I reflect on my forty years of clinical experience, these consultations were fairly straightforward and focused on the medical management of a problem. In the early days of palliative medicine in most medical centers, the palliative medicine consultation focused on symptom management, especially nausea and vomiting and pain. However, we have now emerged into complex discussions on goals of care and decision-making, which can be bewildering for patients and families, especially if the wishes of the patient are not clearly articulated.

Especially as baby boomers age, palliative care will be even more essential. The key point to remember, though, is that it provides a safe harbor in the end-of-life storm, a place of peace and support for patients and their families.

9

How Does Palliative Care Fit?

THE PATIENT, A NINETY-YEAR-OLD NAVY CORPSMAN WHO served in World War II, had fallen in her assisted living apartment and broken her arm. She was admitted to the VA hospital and seemed much more confused than she had been before. Perhaps she had hit her head in the fall too.

With worries about falling and recovery and management of multiple other chronic conditions that involved her heart and long-term back pain, the patient's daughter requested a palliative consult to assess a likely prognosis and offer comfort care. The hospital's social worker was interested because she would help the family find the best next placement—or assess whether the patient could successfully return to assisted living.

The palliative physician sat by the bedside and asked a series of questions to get to know the patient and her wishes, as the daughter silently stood at the foot of the bed, listening.

What they heard was astonishing.

DOCTOR: "What is your understanding of where you are with your illness?"

PATIENT: "Well, I'm here in the hospital, and I broke my arm. This isn't the one I broke when I was twelve and roller-skating, though. How long have I been here?"

DOCTOR: "What are your biggest worries about the future with your health?"

PATIENT: "I don't want to be a burden on my kids. I know it's hard for them. I'll be fine."

DOCTOR: "What aspects of your life are most important to you?"

PATIENT: "Oh, my daughters and their families. My grandchildren and great-grandchildren."

DOCTOR: "Do you think you're dying?" [The palliative doctor wanted her perspective on her situation.]

PATIENT: "No, no, I don't. But I'm ready, you know. My husband died." [Looks at daughter to figure out how long ago; the answer was seven years.]

Most patients respond that they are "going downhill" and say to us, confidentially, "I don't want to tell this to my family." Patients know before the family does, and sometimes it falls to those of us in palliative care to inform the family.

At the end of the assessment, the physician told the daughter that he didn't think her mother was dying, not yet. No palliative measures were needed other than to ease the pain from the broken arm and a chronic back condition. They should be sensitive to the blood thinning medications the patient was taking to prevent stroke and not overmedicate her; they needed to ensure that she did not get dizzy or fall—again.

The VA doctors treated the medical condition, but the palliative specialist looked at the patient and her situation and determined, in this case, that the elderly woman would do just fine in a nursing home with such strong family support nearby.

The confusion might be temporary and possibly from the barrage of pain meds she was taking for the broken arm.

Just because a loved one has broken something, fallen, seems confused, or otherwise seems to be failing, doesn't necessarily mean the worst. A palliative clinician can ask the key questions and interpret the answers in light of the medical situation.

In this case, the hospital's social worker helped the family transition to placement in a nursing home near the daughter, where rehab would take place once the broken arm was healed. Later, she entered a veterans' home and lived another high-quality year and a half.

The healthcare delivery system can be absolutely overwhelming for patients and families. The criticism of the American healthcare system has been well chronicled by multiple journalists, and a recurring theme is that there is no quarterback; patients, when critically ill and especially when hospitalized, are managed by an armada of highly technical subspecialists, many of whom do not know the patient as a person, and families and patients find it difficult to know who their doctor even is.

They ask: Who makes the final decision when it comes to complex medical issues?

It's also becoming clear that a patient's emotional and spiritual needs are often neglected with the rush toward highly invasive and complex interventions, such as cardiac catheterizations and toxic drugs to treat infections, heart failure, and other issues. So where does palliative medicine fit into the big picture?

Practitioners of the subspecialty of palliative care who sit for board certification at this time in history will have had a one-year formal fellowship on the subtleties and nuances of managing patients with complex diseases, like our Navy veteran. Prior to 2012, if physicians had experience dealing with end-of-life patients, they would be automatically eligible to sit for the board exam. However, the restrictions have been significantly tightened, and now individuals who are board eligible in this specialty must have had a twelve-month fellowship.

I am honored to say that I was the first board-certified specialist in palliative and hospice care at Mayo Clinic, and I developed the curriculum for the program in the Mayo Clinic Medical School and was a professor of medicine there, holding a chair as John and Roma Rouse Professor of Humanism in Medicine.

So how does this specialty fit into the big picture for the hospitalized patient facing a terminal illness?

Historically, there has been much confusion about the terms *hospice* and *palliative medicine*. These terms were often used interchangeably and led to considerable confusion not only among patients and families but also among practitioners.

So let me explain. Hospice is a program addressing the social, spiritual, and biological needs of patients with serious illnesses who typically have an expected survival of no more than six months and are no longer seeking treatment for the disease. Two physicians must agree on this timetable, and there are very strict criteria for patients to be enrolled in hospice. There are certain clinical parameters (such as appetite and stamina), as well as biological factors (such as breathing functions and cardiac functions), that determine whether patients are eligible for this Medicare-based benefit.

Expenses related to the patient's illness are largely absorbed by Medicare, but, equally important, patients and families have access 24/7 to credentialed specialists who are trained and comfortable in dealing with symptom management with morphine and other related agents. The hospice program is only a very small percentage of the palliative care community.

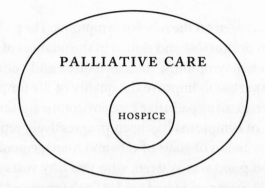

By definition, palliative care, or palliative medicine, is a program of services for patients and families struggling with chronic and life-altering illnesses. The goal and the focus of palliative care is the management of symptoms, the anticipation of complications, and the maintenance of quality of life. Virtually all palliative care organizations would support the following observations about palliative care (and its subcategory of hospice care):

- Palliative specialists affirm life and acknowledge dying as a normal, natural process.

- Neither palliative care nor hospice care hastens or postpones death or prolongs life.

- Such care addresses pain and other symptom management.

- Both embrace and integrate psychological and spiritual aspects of care.

- Practitioners of the specialty enhance a support system so that patients can live as fully as possible and, equally important, offer a support system to families dealing with these difficult and complex issues.

In general, the palliative care consultation service has been asked to see patients usually at the end of life, and, traditionally, the focus had been on the relief of symptoms. The palliative care experts are comfortable and skilled in the nuances of managing pain and other symptoms, such as nausea and vomiting, and have the expertise to improve the quality of life for patients.

However, in many palliative care environments, the emphasis on control of symptoms has been progressively replaced by a broader discussion of goals of care and management.

A case in point was Warren, who was fifty years of age and over an eight-year period had gradually deteriorated from heart failure. He had multiple myocardial infarctions/heart attacks, and the pumping capacity of the heart became significantly compromised. A normal pumping capacity as defined by the ejection fraction is typically about 60 percent. He had an ejection fraction of 5 percent.

Warren had difficult and complex symptoms, including shortness of breath, abdominal distention from fluid (called ascites), and swelling of the lower extremities. Warren was short of breath after only one or two sentences, and his quality of life was not satisfactory to him or to his family.

Traditionally, the palliative care team would be called in to see a patient like Warren literally at the end of life. They would be asked to address the issues of fluid management (checking to see what he was drinking or removing fluid from around his lungs with a procedure), shortness of breath, anxiety, and inability to sleep. Historically, the management of a patient like this primarily focused on medications, but now, with the complexity of illness and the aging of the American population, the focus is quite different.

Many services are now called upon to see patients to address goals of care and also code status. So what do these terms mean?

- *Goals of care* is a broad concept in which there is a thoughtful discussion about the patient's wishes and desires and how these can be framed in a realistic envelope so that goals can be clarified and obtained. Obviously, Warren's hope was for a return to his normal level of functioning, but that goal was not realistic.

- Code status is whether a patient would undergo CPR if the heart stops. This procedure involves shocking the heart with paddle-type devices and, in some circumstances, inserting a breathing tube in the windpipe. Status would be DNR (do not resuscitate) or not.

At this point, I explain to the patient and the family that we have reached a new normal. We cannot turn back the clock, so we need to maximize the patient's quality of life as we now see it. A cure is not on the table. Comfort is paramount. The palliative care team then has the responsibility of refocusing the patient's goals on what is realistic and putting into perspective what is really attainable under the current circumstances.

When queried as to his number-one issue or concern, Warren quickly retorted that he simply wanted to get home with his family, sit on the front porch at his farm, and watch the corn grow. It is this kind of question that the palliative care team typically raises to the patient. What the patient is most concerned about may be far different from the concerns of the primary care team—in this case, the cardiologist.

So the goal of the palliative care team would be to work with the social services community (the hospital's social worker is the main point of contact here) and the patient's local physician to get Warren home so that he could spend his remaining time comfortably with his family and where he wanted to be.

But what if the patient has no family and still wishes to get home? This can be a complex transition involving home health agencies, hospices, and visiting nurse services and requires a major mobilization of resources to acquiesce to and honor the patient's wishes. These transactions are incredibly labor intensive, but they should be in alignment with the patient's wishes.

How and When to Get a Palliative Consult

Like our case at the beginning of this chapter, some families are asking up front for a palliative care consultation early in the patient's hospital stay. It's hard to give a fair percentage on the number of these requests, but there is no doubt that this number continues to increase. So under what circumstances should families, and even patients, ask for a palliative care consultation? And why aren't physicians routinely bringing in palliative colleagues to assist?

Medicine has become so complicated and patients have become so complex that it is the rare patient who will not have a consultation with some subspecialists. Under most circumstances, the primary care physician or the internist admits the patient to the hospital for, let's say, a gastrointestinal hemorrhage. The patient is visited by the gastroenterology service and will undoubtedly have a consultation with the endoscopists who will perform scoping, and the patient may be seen by a surgical consultant, based upon the findings at the scoping. In other words, there are multiple subspecialists brought to the bedside.

Likewise, the palliative care expert has a different perspective on the patient to enhance quality of life and should be part of the care team.

One of my cancer patients, for example, was admitted to the hospital for a serious pneumonia. Sylvia was obviously sick enough to be hospitalized and received high doses of multiple antibiotics under the watchful guidance of the infectious disease team. One of the predictable side effects from her chemotherapy is a condition called peripheral neuropathy. This refers to a very unpleasant burning, lightning-like, crawling discomfort, typically of the hands and feet. While not life threatening, the condition can be disabling in many patients.

Usually, the symptoms are primarily sensory in the form of burning and tingling, but, in some circumstances, there is a motor component where patients may develop a foot drop or have difficulty with fine movement, such as the dexterity required to play cards or handle coins.

In the midst of a major hospitalization like this, the pulmonary team treating the pneumonia obviously does not become distracted with the peripheral neuropathy, even though it's of importance to the patient. So when the palliative care team comes on board, they will be more attuned to that problem and might suggest to the primary care team some medications that may decrease this miserable sensation in the hands and the feet.

Most patients and families are savvy enough to know when they should be seeing a certain subspecialist. If a patient is admitted for pneumonia and then suffers a gastrointestinal hemorrhage, most patients understand that the gastroenterologist would be involved. Likewise, if the patient has multiple symptoms, let's say nausea, vomiting, or pain, which are not being adequately addressed by the primary care team, that would be a situation of bringing to the bedside the palliative care colleague.

So how does this all work? Under most circumstances, the palliative care physician works in tandem with a nurse practitioner or a physician extender. This is typically a master's level individual who would have an RN degree followed by a master's level apprenticeship consisting of approximately 800 hours of careful clinical supervision. These colleagues often make the first contact with the patient, obtain the appropriate history, perform a physical examination, review laboratory studies and imaging interventions, and then present the case to the palliative care consultant, a physician, who then goes to the bedside and repeats the key aspects of the patient's history and physical.

Now, another role of the palliative care team is to act as the quarterback, or the manager, for orchestrating the patient's symptom management when they leave the hospital for home or for a hospice or for a nursing home or a related institution. Under some circumstances, the specific note dictated by the palliative care physician can be lifted off the medical record and shared with the home institution, in terms of medications and dosages and other interventions to enhance quality of life.

Palliative Care at the End of Life

So far, I have explained that palliative does not *necessarily* mean a patient is at the end of life. But now I'm going to circle back and explain how the palliative team assists with end-of-life care.

The palliative team provides specialized care at the end of life that includes relief from symptoms, pain, and the stress of a serious illness—whatever the diagnosis. The goal is to improve quality of life, for both the patient and the family. Some key questions that the palliative care team would raise with the patient are these:

- **What has your doctor told you about your illness?**
  Patients (and family) may respond to this question in a very superficial manner ("Well, Dad doesn't have long to live.") and often don't have an excellent understanding of the situation ("She's having trouble breathing."). The palliative team then knows what the patient and family know and can move ahead to explain the situation ("The breathing problems can be helped with this medication.") and focus on what the patient really needs ("Your dad said he wanted to die at home. What can we do to make that happen?").

- **How do you process information and make decisions?**
  This is also a crucial question. I often ask patients if they want the nitty-gritty medical information or a wider view. We try to judge how much information the patient and family can take in at one time. Do we show scans? Or do we explain in simple terms? Sometimes we draw pictures because even our simple drawings help patients understand

the size of a tumor, for example, in relation to the rest of the liver.

- **What are your biggest worries about the future in terms of your health?**
  What I think the patient should be worrying about may have nothing to do with what the patient is most concerned about. That's why I ask: What are you most fearful about? What keeps you up at night? And the answers can be surprising. Answers include where to die (most choose home) or fear of suffocating (we can address that with medications), but often the focus is on relationships (wanting to see a wayward daughter one more time, eagerness to forgive or acknowledge an illicit relationship, or desire to share a family secret or apologize for financial transgressions).

- **What aspects of your life are most important to you?**
  I try to drill into this issue by saying, "What, if you lost it, would be devastating for you?" Now, think about how you might respond. This could be a loss of dignity or independence or fear of leaving behind someone you love.

If the initial answers to these questions are ambiguous, I simply say, "Tell me more, help me get my arms around this. What do you really mean by XYZ?"

I've also learned the hard way to ask the patient who they would like at the bedside. Sometimes it's a girlfriend rather than the wife. Sometimes it's a same-sex partner the family had suspected but had never really come to grips with.

We on the palliative team are more focused on the patient than on the blood test results or scans.

It's fair for you, as a caregiver, to ask these questions too. Why not? The responses may open once-closed areas of discussion. You'll get a perspective on what the patient is thinking.

10

How Did Palliative Care and Hospice Evolve to Become Such Key Components of End-of-Life Care?

DESPITE THE SPECTACULAR CHANGES IN THE TECHNOLOGY, medications, and delivery of care in the twenty-first century, there is a nagging dissatisfaction among patients and families. The medical care system is viewed as impersonal, not always user friendly or accessible, and many patients and family members are simply distrustful and not pleased with the current predicament. Sound familiar?

Some of this dissatisfaction, coupled with the spiraling cost of healthcare, has placed hospice medicine and palliative care at the forefront of American medicine.

Historically, the major focus on American medicine was to address the acute care crisis—the pneumonia, the heart attack, the trauma patient. But now in America we are faced with a daunting responsibility. Approximately 76 million baby boomers are knocking on the door for healthcare, and managing their care needs has become bewilderingly complicated, with multiple technologies, interventions, and subspecialists—not to mention that the costs are almost unbelievable.

Actually, the costs of care and the issues of access to care, with insurance companies as gatekeepers, are criminal. Simply look at the bill for a routine hospitalized patient: the results are absolutely astonishing.

As discussed, palliative medicine is a subspecialty of internal medicine that focuses on the care of patients with typically chronic or life-threatening illnesses or conditions. Those of us in this specialty work to control symptoms with a bundled approach toward management consisting of the physical aspects of care. We also look at the psychological and psychiatric aspects of care, the social circle around the patient, and the spiritual, religious, and existential aspects of medicine as it relates to a patient. We also address the care of the dying patient.

This concept is relatively new and can be a source of confusion for many patients and families. The training of the specialist consists of four years of medical school, and then, typically two to four years of internal medicine or family practice training, followed by a formal one-year fellowship in an approved palliative care program.

With more than 6,600 board-certified palliative docs among our ranks, you are now likely to find palliative care teams in your local medical centers and hospitals.

Those of us who are board certified pass a grueling ten-hour computer-based exam to show proficiency in the nuances of this specialty. Current manpower estimates suggest that with the aging of the American population and the complexity of care, the optimum number of palliative care specialists needed would be approximately 18,000. And, you are right; we simply don't have that many medical students in the pipeline.

Once upon a time, the palliative care doctor was brought on board at the end of life to control the symptoms of pain, nausea, and vomiting. However, much of our time and efforts and energy are now spent on directions of care and acting as an advocate for the patient and as a translator for the patient and the family, interfacing with a perplexing number of subspecialists. Not all our patients are at the end of life.

Another crucial contribution of palliative care is to share with the patient and the family some understanding of prognosis, either with or without interventions. Without this sort of information, patients and families cannot make reasonably informed decisions. For example, studies now show that when individuals overestimate their prognosis and survival, they are far more willing to undergo complex, sometimes painful and dangerous interventions. On the other hand, when patients understand that their survival is limited, there is far greater willingness to forgo life-sustaining therapies with little meaningful probability of benefit to them.

In general, we specialists recognize that there are developmental tasks that the dying patient must do to achieve peace and serenity. It is the palliative care team, in conjunction with the patient's primary care doctor, that helps facilitate this journey. These major tasks include developing a sense of meaning and purpose, closing the loop on personal events and responsibilities, and bringing closure to earthly affairs, especially in terms of achieving reconciliation and attaining peace.

We practice palliative care in hospitals, in hospice settings that include stand-alone facilities and hospitals, and with patients at home with hospice caregivers.

A Brief History

Let's take a brief look at the history of this program, since there are some important lessons. In the Middle Ages, during pilgrimages and the Crusades, many became ill while traveling or sustained injuries while fighting. Hospices became physical facilities to care for the injured warriors and the ill pilgrims, so the stage was set for caring for people on journeys of all sorts. In the modern concept, the patient's journey is the journey of life and death.

In 1905 the Irish Sisters of Charity started in London and formed St. Joseph's Hospice. This movement was picked up by

Dr. Cicely Saunders, who is now acknowledged as the patron of today's hospice program. She was concerned about the suffering of the dying cancer patient and became instrumental in recognizing and developing the safe use of opiates such as morphine to help these patients during their last days. In 1967 she opened the internationally acclaimed St. Christopher's Hospice in London.

Another crucial development was the 1969 publication of the book *On Death and Dying* by Dr. Elisabeth Kübler-Ross. This book opened the eyes of the community to the needs of the dying patient. It is still a worthy book to read. (After you finish this one, of course!) When Florence Wald, RN, former Dean of Yale University School of Nursing, opened the Connecticut Hospice, the stage was then set for a national presence for this organization in the United States.

Now, a few facts and figures to put this movement into perspective. Up until several years ago, almost 42 percent of all US deaths involved hospice care. Most of this type of care was provided in the patient's home, with a smaller percentage involved in residential facilities or inpatient hospices in hospitals. With the aging of the American population, most hospice patients were in their seventies. Leading diagnoses for hospice patients, as expected, were cancer (35%), heart disease (14%), and dementia (13%).

The Medicare Hospice Benefit

An area of some concern has been the rise of for-profit hospices. Why is this important? Each hospice is designated a fixed per diem amount to care for the patient. Let's say $150. If the patient requires complex interventions and expensive medications, that per diem amount will rapidly be spent. So there has been concern in instances where hospices select patients who would not exceed that per diem. Obviously, there are serious legal and ethical issues with this kind of practice. Although not widely acknowledged, it does cause some concern.

The real challenge is that it's difficult for patients and families to understand what reasonable care is. However, most families can get a sense of what would be appropriate by having an open conversation with the hospice providers to avoid any misunderstandings.

The Medicare hospice benefit applies to a patient whom two physicians—typically the attending physician and a hospice physician—have certified as having an expected prognosis of six months or less. We have guidelines to follow in establishing eligibility for hospice under Medicare, and often we are correct in predicting outcomes. But sometimes we are not right. Sometimes patients do well and live longer than six months. They are then reevaluated and sometimes taken off hospice care.

Current guidelines are these:

1. The patient is eligible for Medicare Part A, meaning the patient is sixty-five years of age or older and receives Medicare payments.

2. The patient has a terminal condition, as determined by two physicians, suggesting a life expectancy of six months or less based on the clinical judgment of the providers.

3. The patient has the informed consent to choose the hospice benefit.

4. The care is provided by a Medicare-certified hospice care program.

From a structural standpoint there are two 90-day periods followed by an unlimited number of 60-day periods. A nurse practitioner must reevaluate the patient, and the hospice physician must certify that the diagnosis and prognosis is appropriate. On occasion, a patient may opt out of the hospice program to seek more aggressive care and then can be readmitted based upon clinical circumstances. After 180 days in hospice, there must be a face-to-face encounter with a hospice physician or nurse practitioner.

Regardless of age, if patients have an expected survival of six months in most circumstances, they are eligible for the Medicare hospice benefit (or are covered by private insurance or charity care).

During times of stress it's certainly predictable that patients and families may not comprehend the subtleties and nuances of the Medicare hospice benefit, so let's just look at this quickly. There are four levels of care:

1. **Routine home care.** This is usually the model where hospice-designated professionals visit the patient, typically several times each week, at home, for a limited period of time (perhaps one or two hours). A common misunderstanding is that a home-based hospice is 24/7 care. Not true. Typically, there is a 24/7 hotline that can be accessed for the hospice nurses, and the family caregivers can call at any time. The hospice team of professionals may include MDs, RNs, social workers, spiritual counselors, bereavement support volunteers, and possibly other services, such as music or massage therapists. These professionals "treat" the patient and the patient's family as a unit.

   This hospice benefit does not cover room and board in a nursing home or hospice facility, and this can be a source of some confusion. If a patient is in a hospice bed in a nursing home, they still receive the hospice benefit, but the room and board fee must be paid by the family.

2. **Continuous home care.** This is when a patient has an acute crisis, such as pain or nausea or vomiting, and there would be intensive home nursing for a minimum of eight hours during each twenty-four-hour period.

3. **General inpatient care.** This is the situation where the patient had been managed at home or in a nursing home, but with an escalation of symptoms has to be temporarily admitted to the hospital or hospice inpatient unit.

4. **Respite care.** There are circumstances where the family/caregivers are completely exhausted, and the patient may be admitted to a facility so that the family can have several days of a break. Most hospices contract with skilled nursing facilities (nursing homes) or use residential hospice for respite care (the patient is transported to the facility).

With the complexity of these programs, it is crucial that there be clear lines of communication among all concerned: the hospice community, the patient's primary care physician, and the hospital. There are circumstances where, in a moment of crisis, the family takes the patient to the emergency room. The patient is hospitalized, and the hospice is not involved. That patient and family may be responsible for an enormous bill. Almost never would a hospice patient need to be whisked to an ER. In fact, caregivers are counseled to call the hospice with all concerns, even 911-type issues.

Getting Answers to Hard Questions

At the end of life, 90 percent of us would choose to receive care in our own homes. However, about 80 percent of us will die in healthcare institutions receiving treatment we don't want. One of the reasons is that there is real misinformation about the hospice program. In general, patients and families often view hospice as a last resort or a sign that they have given up. It's far from that. In fact, with hospice we see overwhelming evidence of enhanced patient satisfaction. In addition, there are significant cost savings.

Another reason why Americans often don't die "at home" depends on geographic location. Seems odd, but data from the *Dartmouth Atlas* showed that 71 percent of people who die in Ogden, Utah, for example, are under hospice care. But only 31 percent are in hospice in Manhattan. If you want to die at home, you might consider living in Sun City, Arizona, where only 12 percent of people die in the hospital.

What factors are at play here? Race is one. African Americans and Hispanics, in my experience, are more reluctant to use the Medicare hospice option because of a general distrust of medicine and a strong family ethos of "we take care of our own." Choice also depends on the doctor. My colleagues who are not as familiar with what we do in palliative care are less likely to recommend such services to their patients.

The choice, perhaps, should be made by the patient and family. I've seen statistics that say less than half of Americans have had a discussion about end-of-life care. It's not the most uplifting topic at the Thanksgiving table. It is my hope that this book encourages more of you to talk about the painful topics around the turkey before one of you is lying in bed and the others are gathered around you.

Let me offer some questions to use as conversation starters. These are adapted from work by Brian Carpenter, a psychologist at Washington University, and Hospice Foundation of America:

- If you had a serious medical issue, such as cancer or stroke or heart attack, what treatments would you want? What would you not want? How would you want your pain handled?

- What decisions regarding care do you want to entrust to others? To whom?

- What aggressive treatments would you want or not want? If treatment isn't curing you, would you stop those treatments?

- Do you want to die at home?

- What do you want to have happen to your body after you die?

- What is most important to you as you approach the end of life, in terms of what you want to accomplish before you die? What do you value most about your life?

These are the kinds of questions that I typically ask patients when we are one-on-one rather than surrounded by a medical entourage. I want to know something about the patient's background and ask them about their legacy. What are they most proud of or wish they could've done over?

Of course, the responses to these questions should be documented on paper in the form of the advance directive, but having the conversation clarifies in the minds of the family—and certainly in the mind of the person designated as the healthcare proxy—what Mom or Grandpa or Aunt Minnie wants. (For an in-depth discussion of the advance directive, see chapters 21 and 22.)

Capacity versus Competence

From my extensive clinical experience in this arena, I have seen a transformation in the position of palliative medicine and hospice care in the management of patients. Our palliative care program at Mayo Clinic started in the late 1990s. When the program was in its infancy, my role primarily focused on symptom management. A small number of us became comfortable with morphine and understood, as did each of our colleagues, the importance of management of such symptoms as nausea, vomiting, and pain.

Over the years, however, our energies have subtly shifted. Many of our discussions now focus on goals of care and the aggressiveness of care or symptom management that patients can access.

Let me share with you a case. Helen was a retired professional in her early eighties who had severe emphysema/COPD. She lived alone in an assisted living facility and took multiple medications. As her disease progressed, she became ensnared in the all-too-familiar cycle of shortness of breath, anxiety, and the midnight trip to the emergency room, followed by intensive management in the hospital, only to be dismissed after several days and then endure a repetition of the cycle.

This pattern of back and forth from hospital to assisted living was frustrating and demoralizing for Helen and her family, and for the caregiving team, and was also frightfully expensive. We on the palliative care service were able to sit down with Helen and her two daughters and suggest an alternative strategy.

She was offered steroid medicines, such as prednisone, and also instructed in the use of morphine, which can decrease shortness of breath. There was a clear understanding that she was not benefiting from these trips to the hospital, and there were clear guidelines on how to manage her symptoms at her living facility with the help of their medical personnel and her daughters.

This program was acceptable to all involved, and Helen peacefully passed away in her own apartment, surrounded by her loving family and neighbors. So in this situation, the palliative care service acted as the translator, as the interpreter, reframing the very appropriate suggestions of the primary care team in the hospital.

Helen was able to help in the decision-making. She was aware of the discussion and knew what she wanted (and didn't want). But an important issue with which we struggle in palliative care is the evaluation of the patient's decision-making capacity when they aren't as aware as Helen was.

There is much confusion in this area. The term *competence* is a legal term; whereas *capacity* really refers to medical treatment decisions. There is an important distinction, especially when we are dealing with issues like transplantation and the use of technologies. In order to have decision-making capacity, patients need to fulfill a number of criteria, which we can easily assess at the bedside:

- Can express insight of the situation; can clearly and consistently articulate the diagnosis and prognosis and the pros, cons, risks, and options of treatment

- Can make a rational choice based on personal issues

- Is not delusional or in the midst of an untreated psychiatric disease

- Shows a firm preference and does not vacillate

Over time, patients may *not* have competence in, say, investing in the stock market, but they may have clear capacity when it comes to medical decisions.

To provide some support during these difficult decisions, such organizations as the American Academy of Hospice and Palliative Medicine have offered policy statements. They make it quite clear when considering nonbeneficial interventions. In other words, whether these interventions are not started or are withdrawn is morally the same.

Let's focus on the issue of renal (kidney) dialysis, for example. This is a complex intervention where a procedure called a fistula is performed. This typically involves accessing a large vein in the arm. The patient undergoes a filtering of the blood, typically three times a week for four or five hours. After the dialysis, most patients feel generally unwell and confused. Almost never will the patient undergoing dialysis feel better from the procedure. It's at moments like these that, if the patient has capacity and wishes to discontinue the dialysis, ceasing (withdrawing) the treatment will be the morally appropriate thing to do.

Betty had kidney failure for years. She made three trips a week to the dialysis center miles from her home in a small town. By age seventy-nine, she decided she had lived a good life. She was tired of the procedures. She didn't always feel "well."

She completely understood her decision, made in consultation with her family doctor, to enter the local nursing home's hospice program, discontinue dialysis, and quietly die, on her own terms, within days. And that's what she did.

Betty eventually felt herself slipping away. The medications her doctor ordered to make her comfortable were begun. The atmosphere in the hospice suite was subdued at times and teary (but not without festivity; empty beer bottles and popcorn were cleaned up by housekeeping staff one morning).

Barbara, on the other hand, at age ninety-two, was unable to express her wishes. When she had capacity some months earlier, she had filled out an advance directive naming her son as healthcare proxy. She wanted no heroic measures taken. She was living in a veterans' home, on the nursing care wing. When she became obviously short of breath, unable to speak or make sense, and had to lean over to try to get her breath because of severe complications from advancing and irreversible congestive heart failure, her son said, "Let's call in palliative and hospice, start the morphine, and get her into bed."

Her death the next morning was expected. She spent her last night tucked into bed, in her own pajamas, with her son at her side, holding her hand and having a one-sided conversation about how wonderful her life had been. At that point, Barbara didn't have capacity or competence. Her disease was calling the shots, along with her devoted son, who followed the advance directive.

A key assessment is the capacity of the patient—or the substituted judgment of the patient's surrogate or proxy—as to whether or not the patient would want a particular intervention. In these examples, either the patient or the proxy made the decisions. No calls to 911. No chest compressions for CPR. No last-minute what-ifs, no looking back.

11
What Is Hospice?

LET'S TALK ABOUT A TOPIC THAT NO ONE REALLY WANTS TO address, but if we ignore it, we do so at our peril. This is the hospice program.

There is tremendous confusion among patients, families, and even healthcare providers regarding this concept. We cannot really address hospice without some acknowledgment of palliative care, and this has been an ongoing theme so far in this book.

In short, the palliative medicine program nationwide focuses on quality of life, sense of well-being, and addresses the biological, psychological, emotional, social, and spiritual needs of patients and families. It is life affirming. It is not supportive of physician-assisted suicide or euthanasia.

Historically, palliative medicine was brought on toward the end of life to enhance symptom management, but there is an emerging and consistent trend in the cancer community that palliative care has moved "upstream" upon the diagnosis of cancer and becomes more robust and more involved in patient care as the disease progresses.

The hospice dimension is a very small sliver of the palliative medicine pie. As my colleague, Beverly Haynes, the executive director of Seasons Hospice, and a nurse herself, pointed out so gently in the writing of this book, "Hospice is a philosophy of care, accepting death as a normal part of life."

In simplistic terms, hospice is a Medicare-derived benefit that is typically utilized when patients have an expected survival of six months or less. We've touched on this already, but let me emphasize that this is not a rigid rule. Your healthcare providers need to ask themselves one question: "Is it more likely than not that the patient will die of their condition within six months?" If the answer is yes, that patient is eligible for the hospice benefit.

Under most circumstances, a patient is evaluated by the hospice medical director, in concert with one of their designates, who is typically a nurse or a physician extender. There are relatively straightforward and sometimes unreasonably rigid criteria for patients to be admitted to hospice.

At one time, the guidelines were relatively loose, and some patients would be involved or enrolled in a hospice program for years. For example, if the patient has end-stage congestive heart failure, they must meet certain criteria to be eligible. This would include the ejection fractions that measure the pumping function of the heart, as well as the patient's overall sense of strength and stamina.

Patients with heart or lung disease must meet certain criteria in terms of the EKG and echocardiogram results and other parameters in order to be eligible for hospice. Likewise, if patients have dementia or an Alzheimer's-like illness, there are clear benchmarks. In other words, if a patient is not eating well, is unable to walk, is incontinent, or is unable to speak a certain number of intelligent words in a sentence, that patient may be eligible for hospice.

You don't have to know these criteria. That's the responsibility of the medical care team. But there needs to be a general awareness that simply "not doing well" does not automatically make a patient a hospice candidate.

The bottom line is that if the reasonably anticipated trajectory of the patient's illness would suggest that the patient will die within six months, that patient may well be eligible for the hospice benefit. And now I'm back to saying we doctors don't play God—even though actors play God as doctors on TV—and we don't know how long someone may live. We just don't.

Types of Hospice Settings

Generically speaking, there are two forms of hospice:

- **A home-based program.** Certified hospice clinicians, who are typically nurses with advanced training, visit the patient several times each week for approximately one hour to assess symptoms, regulate medications, assist with personal care and hygiene, interact with family members as to the patient's course, and have a hands-on as well as a 30,000-foot view of the patient's issues. Focus is on bowel, bladder, and pain, as well as sleep and other concerns.

  If the patient is deteriorating or if there is a major change in medication needed, the hospice nurse, who really is the "boots on the ground," will then connect with the hospice medical director or the patient's personal physician.

  One of the key aspects of the home-based program is that the family has a phone number to call should they be concerned about the patient's condition. Otherwise, without hospice support, it is very difficult to contact the appropriate individual who can address the patient's and the family's concerns at any hour of the day or night.

  Most hospices, which are home-based, do require a caregiver to be in the home, although this is not a rigid rule. Obviously, if the patient is profoundly disabled, a home-based program may not be reasonable.

  "Home" in this sense is wherever the patient calls home, which could be a private home, a daughter's home, a nursing home, or assisting living, for example.

- **The bricks-and-mortar hospice facility.** In some communities, this is a homelike setting, hotel-type environment, or a private home that has been modified for patients with terminal illness. Under some circumstances, there are designated hospice beds in a nursing home or in an acute care hospital where the patient's needs are met outside the home.

The patients are in a safe and secure environment where the focus is on quality of life and sense of well-being, and there is the clear understanding that there is not a focus on high-tech invasive interventions, such as radiation therapy and chemotherapy and blood transfusions, since these often do not enhance quality of life. Nevertheless, there are circumstances where these interventions might be appropriate even in the dying patient, and these must be addressed on an individual basis.

In most hospices, there are liberal visiting hours, and family members and patients have the right to receive compassionate care and to have their questions addressed and resolved in a timely and respectful manner.

Some patients have complex needs that cannot be met in a home-based facility, so a hospice-designated bed in a convalescent/nursing home or in a hospital would best suit that patient's needs. The alternative is a hospice "house." There are obvious advantages to that situation, but a major disadvantage that many patients verbalize is that it is not "home." Hospice facilities can be comfortably "homelike," with kitchens and showers available for family caregivers, bedside sleeping chairs, a chapel, snacks, and caring staff 24/7. The family pets are often welcome.

Most of my patients express a desire to die at home. However, this is often not possible, especially when there are complex medical needs or if there is a significant pain problem that needs close monitoring by a medical team. If the caregiver of the patient is elderly and/or infirm, home is simply not a workable option.

And Now a Little Insight

Products compete with one another to be the best: books vie to become best sellers; restaurants claim to have the best meatloaf; and now well-publicized national registries are pitting healthcare delivery systems against each other. Why are some hospitals ranked number one for orthopedic surgery or in the top ten for cancer care or some other measure?

It's about marketing, of course. And when patients die in the hospital, guess who keeps track? A host of government agencies and ranking organizations. Most medical practitioners won't tell you about this dark secret, but I will.

In general, if there is a death in the hospital within thirty days of admission or within thirty days of surgery, this goes "against" a healthcare system. Facetiously, no one dies within thirty days of surgery, and this is why many postoperative patients are supported to pass that thirty-day mark. It measures nothing. All cases and patients are different.

But there is an emerging movement that if a patient dies on hospice care in the hospital, this does not "count" in the death column. Therefore, if a patient is a hospice candidate and if within thirty days of hospitalization, the administrative machinery gears up to enroll that patient in hospice, the patient is moved to a separate wing or floor or room and is considered a hospice patient.

The good news is that patients get excellent end-of-life care, from me and from teams like ours. On the other hand, some families have felt pressured—or, should I say, they felt gently pushed—into the hospice arena without a lot of planning and discussion. Just be aware, you have options, and you don't have to stay in that hospital if you are feeling pressured. And now you know your loved one may be viewed as an unwanted statistic—an unfortunate development that my colleagues and I are not happy about.

The option to choose one hospice setting or the other is profoundly personal. Some individuals have had negative experiences of friends and family members dying at home, and for that individual, the bricks-and-mortar facility may be more ideal.

In hospice settings, there is a clear understanding that death is the result of natural causes or the evolution of an underlying process. Consequently, the goal of the hospice program is to alleviate psychological, emotional, spiritual, and physical suffering—not to hasten death.

12

Why Is the Family Meeting So Critically Important?

THE PATIENT WAS AN EDUCATOR AND A PROMINENT administrator from a small Midwestern community college. Richard had struggled with black mole cancer, malignant melanoma, which had spread from his foot into the abdominal area and then into multiple lymph nodes. In January, he developed multiple spots in the brain (central nervous system metastasis). These were treated with whole brain radiation therapy, and he did well for several months.

But when he returned in May to see me, the lymph nodes, which contained cancer in the abdomen, were more prominent, and Richard was subtly confused. His *executive functioning* was impaired. You might hear this term. In other words, he was unable to make decisions or follow through on making reasonable choices. He could not process information in a meaningful and reasonable way. This type of confusion involves the brain's frontal lobes, which can often be damaged because of dementia or lack of oxygen.

In addition, his gait was unstable. All these findings strongly suggested growth of the tumorous nodules in the brain. And this was confirmed with an MRI scan.

Richard had previously received several types of chemotherapy, which clearly were not working, so we were now faced with the distressing dilemma of where to go from here. What does the future hold? What are the options?

In circumstances such as these, patients cannot be expected to retain or absorb or process the information received from the medical team. We had anticipated that the patient would not be totally engaged, but at the time of the consultation, Richard was accompanied by his adult daughter and his two brothers.

Each medical professional has a toolbox. The neurologist has a reflex hammer in his toolbox. The cardiologist has a stethoscope in her toolbox. The surgeon has a scalpel. A crucial tool in the box of the palliative care specialist is that of the family meeting.

I start these discussions by calling the family together. The family conference is typically held in a quiet room *without the patient being present,* although the patient may be made aware the meeting is occurring. Once the family reaches consensus about the direction of care, we would all go to the bedside for a review with the patient. It is awkward to have that meeting in a hospital setting, but you may find family members gathered around the bedside and a doctor and medical team in deep discussion.

For out-of-towners, such as family members who have yet to show up, we set up speakerphones. Invited are the key players of the care team: the physicians, the physical therapist, the registered dietitian, the chaplain, the nurses, and other major partners in the patient's care. This is crucial so that everyone is on the same page and there are no misunderstandings.

Typically, the palliative care person directs the conversation with the family. I often ask this: "From what you have seen so far, how do you anticipate this illness playing out? What do you think might be occurring over the next several weeks or months?"

Each team member identifies themselves, and each member of the family is asked to relate what the team has told them. It is crucial that clear time boundaries be set. Let's say forty-five minutes, and then the professional team will exit and leave the family behind for further discussion.

In the case of Richard's cancer, I clearly explained that our options were limited. There were no curable interventions, but there were types of chemotherapy that could be considered. The surgeon said there were no reasonable surgical options. The family raised reasonable questions about the pros, cons, risks, and benefits of each treatment and were able to support the patient's wishes not to proceed with additional treatment options.

It is important for family members to be engaged in this critical discussion so that there is a clear understanding of the decision-making process. The role of the palliative care expert in this setting is to act as a translator by reframing and putting into perspective the bewildering amount of clinical information.

If it is consistent with the wishes of the patient and the family, it is often helpful for us to review the actual images themselves. I can show a CT scan on the hospital's computer screens and point out areas of concern. Sometimes seeing the problem goes a long way toward helping the patient and family members understand the progression of the disease. But an important warning: I always ask the patient and family if they wish to see the pictures. On occasion, these can be so markedly abnormal that it is very upsetting to everyone. You may also ask to see images if they are not offered.

Another important dimension of the family conference is for the palliative care team to affirm and be supportive of the family's collective decision. There is nothing more anguishing for patients and families than to look backward and ask the "if only" questions: "If only we had just done X or Y, the outcome would be different." This is a heavy burden. Feel reassured that you have done the right thing. And there is little merit in looking back, since that consumes an enormous amount of wasted energy.

Ultimately, there was clear agreement that Richard was not a candidate for additional treatment, but the dots were still not connected. There was still unfinished business. The patient was a widower. He had been living alone in a multilevel home, and this clearly was not a safe situation. At that point, the conversation went in a new direction: how best to give Richard quality of whatever life he had remaining. And his family set to the task with renewed hope and optimism.

In another case, Erin's father was in the ICU, where he never regained consciousness after a serious downturn in his condition. She shares the end-of-life outcome we all hope for every family in these situations: "Family was there every day, and we had a lot of support from the doctors, nurses, and hospital social worker. While it was a wretched experience, I feel like we did it the right way: we made decisions as a family, supported each other, spent time with Dad, and made the best decision for him that we could."

What Happens When the Family Cannot Agree?

Another dimension of the expertise of the hospice and palliative care community is dealing with the family when there is a striking divergence of opinion on care management.

Joaquin, a gentleman in his late forties, developed an infection of the heart called a viral myocarditis. This dramatically impaired the pumping chamber of the heart, and he evolved into congestive heart failure punctuated by profound shortness of breath and massive swelling of the abdomen and legs. Despite every appropriate medical intervention, his heart continued to fail, and the only approach of any potential value was a left ventricular assist device.

At one point in history, these were viewed as a bridge to sustain the patient prior to heart transplantation, but with the diminishing number of transplantable hearts available, these mechanical devices are now viewed as "destination therapy"— meaning therapy in and of itself.

These incredibly complex surgical procedures can clearly enhance quality of life and length of life in some patients—those who can get through the initial month or so following surgery, where there is a high risk of bleeding, blood clots, and infection.

In our particular patient, the situation continued to deteriorate because the mechanical pumping devices became infected. He developed liver and kidney failure, so he required dialysis, and we reached a point where it was unlikely that Joaquin would ever leave the hospital in a functioning status.

Now let's look at his psychosocial history, which is absolutely crucial. He was a prominent businessman in a small community. He had two adult children from an initial marriage that resulted in divorce, and now had a second family of a wife and three young children. The patient himself was conflicted as to the aggressiveness of care. His second wife insisted that everything possible be done, while his parents basically said, "Enough is enough. Let's stop everything and focus on comfort measures."

This sort of family conflict is all too common and requires a skillful clinician to acknowledge and honor everyone's wishes to help the patient make the appropriate decision.

We in the palliative community have learned through painful experiences that there are no shortcuts. There are no quick fixes, and one way to address this issue of how aggressively to continue care is with a family conference (with or without the patient present).

I've already described the meeting in generic terms. Let me now emphasize that, during the meeting, there is typically a cascade of feelings and emotions and often hidden agendas among multiple family members. At the end of the meeting, a bottom line is quite clear to those family members present when the answer to this question is considered: "What is the best decision for the patient's well-being, rather than what decision do I, as a family member, want for the patient?" We as clinicians are mindful to separate our wishes and our desires from that of the patient too.

I personally am often astounded at the lengths and the discomfort that patients will go through when the probability of a positive outcome is vanishingly small and the suffering brought upon the family can be devastating. I recall one patient, a relatively young man with a failing heart. He was completely hooked up to just about every mechanical device we had. He was not a candidate for a heart transplant. The first wife and kids and the second wife and kids had moved to Rochester and were living in an extended stay motel. For weeks. There was no probability that he would ever get better, yet he still had capacity to insist on every possible medical intervention we had.

But with Joaquin and his family, we discussed clear milestones. For example, if his weight did not increase by five pounds within the next two weeks, we would need to seriously think about discontinuing the aggressiveness of management. If the fever did not resolve with these strong antibiotics and if he could not be up and about for half of his waking hours, this was a sign that we should consider winding down on some of these aggressive interventions.

In other words, no one "pulls the plug"—which is sort of a Hollywood euphemism, anyway—but there is a clear discussion about measurements or milestones that need to be reached to tell us about the relative futility of continuing some of these measures.

If you are faced with these types of agonizing decisions, it's important to engage the patient in these discussions so that there is complete transparency of the decision-making process. I'm reminded of the all-too-typical scenario where we on the care team have a serious end-of-life discussion around the bedside with the patient and the family. We then walk into the hallway and are followed by a parade of family members who say, "Okay, Doc, tell me what's really going on."

When this occurs, the medical team respectfully returns to the room so that the patient understands there are no "hidden deals" and all the facts are clearly on the table. Not only is this the right thing to do, but also, in virtually every medical center, patients have complete access to their records, and it can be devastating for the patient to read something in the record contrary to what the primary care team shared with that patient.

The family meeting is typically held every five days. In Joaquin's case, he did not thrive. His wife finally agreed that aggressive measures were not working, although we had tried.

And then there's this scenario: Harrison made a fortune in commercial real estate. His wife was equally prominent in their Midwestern city. He came to me as a patient, and I to his bedside as he was admitted with major complications from his prostate cancer. The couple's three grown sons accompanied them. I don't know what their family dynamics were like growing up, but these boys argued with their mother, talked back to their father, sniped at each other, and I was concerned about having to call hospital security if the arguments escalated to shoving and punching.

As it turns out, the anger these *children* showed in the presence of their father's dire circumstances naturally turned to me—to the limitations of modern medicine, to the unknowns about various courses of treatment, to why couldn't we cure their father, and on and on.

I could offer no guarantees for Harrison, but these boys were certain the cure for their father's situation was on the internet—as if we at the Mayo Clinic were keeping the secret cure under wraps. They had their laptops and had performed Google searches and read about miracles in third-world countries and unsupported medical accounts. They had not navigated to credible medical journals or visited the medical library. But now that they were "experts," they wanted to dictate the course of treatment. They posed question after question about a drug they had read about or a technique in some foreign country or a supplement "guaranteed" to make a miracle happen.

In our family meetings, they kept asking, "What about this?" "What about that?" "Have we thought about this?" Asking the same questions and hoping for a different answer, while wasting valuable time that should have been spent on helping their father.

We on the medical team give our patients our best advice and work with the patients to honor their wishes and guide the next treatment step (knowing that sometimes that next step may be no treatment at all). But when family members—in this case, three angry adult men—bring belligerence and aggression to the family meeting, those of us in the white coats find it very difficult to work in these situations.

I will confide this to you: We often push back in these confrontational settings. Not that we'd go along with another MRI just because Junior plays doctor and thinks Dad needs one, but we cringe in horror at the family dynamics, the one-upping, and choose to remove ourselves from the soap opera playing out over the deathbed. We are reluctant to engage in medical conversations involving outrageous cures and internet promises. Time is better spent talking with Dad about his hopes and expectations, relieving his pain and suffering, not indulging a know-it-all kid (or adult) with a laptop and Wi-Fi.

If the odd man out is not one of the patient's children, it's a grandson or a well-meaning church member who had a "similar cancer" or a distant relative who flies to the bedside, bringing a cloud of gloom and doom and demands that the medical team "fix this." So you can imagine how some of these contentious family meetings play out.

The fix is this: Families are counseled to choose a quarterback if that person is not the patient. We encourage discussion around what's best for Dad or Grandma. When everyone is focused on that goal, these meetings often find consensus and a path forward with less drama.

Perhaps once or twice a week, families will ask me if they could record (the audio) of the consultation. With some reluctance, I agree. The problem is that this forces me to measure and weigh every comment, and it really eliminates some of the humanity of a consultation. Not that I would misspeak or find these audio conversations played back in court at a malpractice suit. But I am, like everyone, a little more cautious when a recorder or smartphone comes between the holy sanctity of the conversation between my patient and me.

A new wrinkle in the recording of these encounters comes when someone asks if the conversation could be FaceTimed or Skyped and streamed to family members in Timbuktu. I draw the line on this intrusion, under the umbrella of patient confidentiality. I carefully explain that if the stream is intercepted, the video could go viral with tremendous consequences, and I've never really been challenged on this point.

When Hospice Might Be Considered

In Joaquin's case, the treatment didn't go well. At some point the family meeting included discussion of where he would go next. Staying in the hospital is not often an option because other stakeholders around the bed get involved. And I'm talking about the insurance company. We are pressured to dismiss (or move) patients earlier than in past decades. Any escalation in care in the hospital would not be covered. Sadly, patients and their families are often forced to make care decisions based on coverage.

We on the palliative team have options in our lab coat pockets. Rather than coming out and recommending a hospice intervention, I often ask this: "Have you considered the hospice alternative?"

This terminology is helpful, since the word *hospice* can have a negative connotation in certain circumstances. In some settings, the term is associated with giving up or closing chapters, and it can also be equated with leaving the patient isolated in some sort of facility. Family members with this type of mind-set about hospice might respond by saying something like this: "We're just sending Mom off to die, right?"

This is an excellent opportunity to open the discussion with the medical team on the Medicare hospice benefit and what it actually involves. There are profound misunderstandings about how hospice works.

It is during the family meeting that I can explain that, in most communities, a hospice is a home-based program where credentialed, certified healthcare providers touch base with the patient, typically for an hour or so and typically for several days each week. It is important to emphasize that this is a 24/7 service with access to an RN and acts as a conduit or connection between the patient and the hospice medical director and the patient's primary care physician.

Some hospice programs offer an option of staying in a hospice facility, with private or semiprivate rooms. Or being treated as a hospice patient while living in a nursing home. And there are emergency hospice options, both in stand-alone facilities and within hospital settings for short-term stays when a patient is referred there from an emergency room, usually when a medical condition worsens to the point where the family cannot take care of the patient at home. The patient may then be transitioned to home or back to home.

We underscore that patients and families cannot be expected to understand if a symptom or a complaint is serious or a trivial inconvenience. There is a hotline so that families can connect with a hospice professional to sort out the urgency of a concern.

In my own experience, the hospice benefit has been of great value for patients and families because it often allows the patient to remain at home during some difficult times. A comment that I commonly hear goes something like this: "The hospice nurses were absolutely wonderful. I'm only sorry that we were not aware of this benefit early in Dad's illness."

I can tell you from personal experience with family members and from comments by patients and their families every day that the hospice nurse is a special human being described by these attributes: extremely caring, highly professional, knowledgeable about the dying process, reassuring to the family, always accessible, and respectful of decisions. The hospice nurse provides a shoulder to cry on, an understanding bedside manner, a reassuring voice on the phone at 3:00 a.m., and a comforting presence when the entire end-of-life process seems overwhelming.

Hospice offers a caring option when patients and families can thoughtfully discuss and select the next step.

13

What Is Patient-Centered Management at the End of Life?

DR. MARCUS WELBY RETIRED YEARS AGO. EVEN MY OWN FAMILY doctor, Dr. Frank, and his colleagues stopped making house calls when Eisenhower was president. Medicine today is far different from what our parents experienced. Heck, medicine has evolved immensely during my tenure as a physician, and I continue to be astounded and delighted at the advances in care, especially some enormous steps in cancer treatment and cure. (Yet, like most physicians, I am disappointed in access to care and how insurance companies, politics, and Big Pharma get between me and my patients. That is a sensitive topic playing out in political circles even as I write this.)

Medicine traditionally had been a paternalistic, almost dictatorial profession. Physicians were educated. They were prominent in the community, and their word was accepted as gospel. No debate. No discussion. You simply did whatever the doctor said. Even today, your aging mother may simply know that the doctor prescribed the little yellow pills "for her heart," and she takes them faithfully, with a glass of water, every morning. Am I right?

This doctor-as-God model evolved in the Middle Ages when patients were relatively uneducated and obviously had virtually no concept of medical or biological theories—nor did the doctors, for that matter. With the evolution of the printing press and the education of the masses, this situation started to slowly change and skyrocketed with easy access to health websites.

Now the pendulum has dramatically shifted 180 degrees. Patients have become more empowered. And the patient—rightfully so—is the focus of the decision-making process. In an ideal world, the patient, the family, and the doctor have a collaborative relationship.

So let's look at an example of how this can work.

Susan, a fifty-something woman, a small business owner, had a previous history of lung cancer, which was surgically treated for cure, and no chemotherapy or radiation was necessary. When she returned to see me for follow-up visits, scans and bloodwork were clear (in fact, one of her cancer markers in her blood was quite low), but an unusual swelling in her neck signaled something was going on.

We discovered an enlarged lymph node. It turned out to be a new primary cancer of the ovary, and she underwent chemotherapy and suffered many of its nasty side effects. Needless to say, the chemotherapy experience was not particularly pleasant. However, what was encouraging was that staging scans and assessments at the end of the chemotherapy sessions showed no active evidence of cancer.

Following usual guidelines, Susan returned at quarterly intervals for routine evaluations with scans, cancer-related blood tests, as well as a careful history and physical examination. For approximately seven months after discontinuing chemotherapy, she did amazingly well.

But during one follow-up, we discovered another swollen lymph node near her heart. She was concerned and anxious but had zero enthusiasm to go through the chemotherapy treatment once again and felt quite comfortable to return for additional evaluations.

At this point everyone—the patient, her husband, and two sons—were in agreement that we did not have to become overwhelmingly concerned, but a reassessment in three months was the appropriate thing to do.

During the next follow-up, the lymph node had enlarged. Since it was highly likely and highly probable that this lymph node harbored cancer, early in my career there would have been a firm recommendation for chemotherapy, with very little debate or discussion. In a sense, the patient would have been clearly told what to do. Her concerns would have been acknowledged, but the patient almost always went along with the medical recommendation. In this case, it would have been for chemotherapy.

But now let's look at the situation through the lens of contemporary medicine, through the lens of the patient-physician relationship, through the lens of the shared decision-making process.

Susan made it quite clear that even if the lymph node did harbor cancer, she did not want chemotherapy. So, with this in mind, there really was no reason to subject the patient to the risks and the complications of a biopsy, since, even if it did show cancer, she was not interested in further treatment. Heresy? No, an empowered patient.

These are not the kinds of discussions that anyone wants to have late in the doctor's day or at the end of a busy clinic in the morning. No patient should feel rushed. The doctor and patient need to carefully examine the options, and in the end, the patient's wishes win out—a far cry from doing what the doctor says, no questions asked.

Family members need to be respectful of the wishes of the patient, even though the patient's decision may be at odds with the decision that other family members would make.

It is also vitally important during these emotionally charged issues that responsible family members act as a filter or a translator or an interpreter, to reframe or clarify the comments of the healthcare provider. It is apparent that during a charged emotional encounter relating to cancer, patients don't always retain all the facts or even remember most of the conversation. Someone with a smartphone may record the conversation, or someone else in the room may take notes.

These sorts of decisions are made even more complicated because almost without exception patients access their issues on the internet and they read their medical records and often keep copies. A Google search can be helpful but more often than not profoundly misleading. Many healthcare organizations give patients a portal to access their own medical records and diagnostic studies, but I caution that without proper interpretation from a healthcare provider, patients may feel frustrated, alarmed, and confused about their results.

The Empowered Patient, the Informed Family

As medicine evolves to become more patient-centered and family-centered, rather than physician-centered, major medical organizations including the American Board of Internal Medicine and its nonprofit foundation have issued guidelines entitled "Choosing Wisely." This is a very aggressive and robust educational program to empower patients and families to work with their healthcare providers to avoid unnecessary and dangerous recommendations.

Let me share the five interventions that patients, their families, and healthcare providers should challenge each other on when it comes to bedside care of a loved one. These topics often drive the family meeting discussions:

1.   There can be a collaborative, tandem relationship between the palliative care provider and the doctors offering disease-specific treatment. A landmark study by our colleagues at Massachusetts General Hospital involved patients with advanced lung cancer. Each received standard chemotherapy, and half were randomly allocated to also receive aggressive

palliative care treatment. The group receiving palliative therapy with chemotherapy outlived the other patients by about three months. So palliative medicine can provide a valuable adjunct while disease-specific therapy is in place.

2. As physicians, we do not push for feeding tubes in patients with dementia, but we do focus on oral assisted feeding. Overwhelming evidence from multiple centers throughout the world clearly document the risks and the complication of these devices with little short- or long-term benefit. I discuss feeding tubes in more detail elsewhere, but suffice it to say, the decision to insert a feeding tube is not one to be made casually.

3. If the patient and family are comfortable with and embrace a palliative symptomatic care trajectory, it does not make sense to leave in place an implantable cardioverter-defibrillator to be activated, which can shock the patient and provide no meaningful benefit. Let's have these discussions up front rather than at 2:00 a.m. and under dire circumstances.

4. Patients and family should understand that large, peer-reviewed studies now document that if a patient has a painful bone lesion from advanced cancer, one fraction— one "shot"—of radiation may be as effective and certainly far more convenient than the traditional program that typically had consisted of treatments for five days a week for three consecutive weeks.

5. Topical gels and lotions, while appealing, offer very little benefit for treating nausea caused by chemotherapy. The use of lorazepam (Ativan), diphenhydramine (Benadryl), and Haldol as gels for alleviating nausea has become trendy, but these approaches are no more effective than orally administered medicines.

So these guidelines and more are clearly underscoring that patients and families need to be engaged, need to be knowledgeable, and need to partner with the medical team to receive reasonable, optimal care—especially toward the end of life.

There's Always Hope

Even if we run out of options or medications, I always offer the one medicine in my bag that never goes away: hope.

Hope has a variety of definitions, but from a medical standpoint, hope is the expectation that a situation will turn out as best as it possibly can. Many of us have learned over the years that hope is not a fixed destination but a moving target. Let me explain.

Upon the diagnosis of a serious problem, most patients naturally expect and hope for a cure and a return to normal functioning. Stephanie noticed a rapid pulse. She felt generally well but did not want to ignore this situation. Her father had died of heart issues, and now, at sixty-eight, she was concerned about her genetic destiny.

She saw her primary care doctor, who also noticed a rapid pulse and the absence of any other developments. This was confirmed by an electrocardiogram, which showed no heart muscle damage but did confirm a pulse of about 110, compared with a normal pulse of about 80. The primary care physician appropriately performed an echocardiogram, which consists of putting a microphone-type device over the breastbone. The results were stunningly shocking: her heart was pumping at about half of its capacity, and to make up for this deficit, the heart was working overtime, accounting for the rapid pulse.

A referral to a cardiologist was in order, and it appeared that Stephanie had suffered an unusual viral infection of the heart, which caused a weakening of the heart muscle. So upon hearing this news, her first hope was for a cure, some medication, or some intervention to fix the problem.

As the months evolved, it became clear that there was no simple solution. There was no cure, and at this point she switched hope from the target of a cure to the target of adaptation and adjustment and acclimation to the situation. As the shortness of breath and fatigue became more troublesome, she realized the importance of budgeting her energies—bundling routine tasks and errands, curtailing late-night social activities as well as alcohol usage, and being more mindful of rest and time for meditative reflection.

The next stage in this journey of hope was the recognition that the condition was deteriorating and now was the time to connect the dots, to circle the wagons, and to close those painful chapters and cross bridges of healing, peace, serenity, and reconciliation.

Stephanie had the gift to recognize that what we hope for at the start of a diagnosis may be very different from what we hope for as the journey unfolds. Interestingly, one of the "gifts" she shared with me was that this heart problem was a stimulus, an incentive to recognize that she had more sand at the bottom of the hourglass than in the top of the hourglass. It was time to swallow pride and reach out to her sister, with whom there had been a strained and painful relationship.

She never gave up hope; she just redefined her definition of it.

14

When Do We Start and Stop Medication?

A KINDLY GRANDMOTHER FROM FARGO WAS IN OUR HOSPICE service because she was dying of heart failure. She had a cascade of medical conditions, and the outcome was certain, but one troubling development was dehydration. It was certainly appropriate to provide her with a quart of intravenous fluids. This is sometimes controversial, but, in this situation, it was the right thing to do.

After receiving approximately two-thirds of the IV fluids, she became increasingly fatigued and simply wanted to be left alone. She told us so. And she also told her four sons gathered around the hospital bed. One of the first rules in medicine is to honor the wishes of the patient and recognize that it is not all about us, but about the patient and the family. So we disconnected the IV, and she was able to sleep restfully—a win-win situation for everyone.

One essential dimension of palliative medicine is to step back and be realistic about when to start and stop medications. For example, if a patient is young and relatively healthy and has experienced major trauma, such as an automobile accident or some combat-related issue, meticulous attention to medical details is obviously crucial, specifically in regard to dosages and timing of medications.

But if a patient is at the end of life and the major focus is on comfort and control of symptoms, we need to acknowledge some wiggle room. For example, for a dying patient on blood thinners to prevent a stroke, measuring the levels through blood testing is not critical at all, nor is it even prudent to continue to give a dying patient statins to lower their cholesterol when their lifespan is limited to a number of weeks. Or to continue vitamins or osteoporosis meds, not to mention many other meds, including blood pressure meds that can often cause light-headedness.

When it comes to antidepressants for patients at the end of life, they are fine for someone who has been on them over time, but to start these medications that don't kick in for four to six weeks isn't realistic.

Same with diet. Why would anyone want to deprive a dying patient of ice cream or a special treat or continue a low-fat, low-salt diet? These are some of the few pleasures patients may have. I still cringe when I see seriously ill patients smoking in the designated areas of the hospital. I understand the addiction. But that is their choice, and I respect it.

Now let's focus for a moment on blood draws and imaging interventions. These are never pleasant experiences. Who wants to lie still for yet another MRI or get poked by the phlebotomists for more vials of blood? And we need to ask ourselves and the patient why are we doing what's being suggested. Will the outcome of this blood study or this scan make any meaningful difference in the management of the patient? If the result will not change the overall clinical care, then perhaps the test should not be performed at all.

Also note that once a patient is on hospice, Medicare and most insurance will no longer cover the cost of these interventions, so deciding whether to have imaging or testing should be for practical symptom management, because the treatment decision has already been made.

Family members certainly have the appropriate right, in concert with the patient, to inquire about the pros and cons and risks and benefits of a specific medication or procedure or scan or blood test (even if the monitors need to be hooked up at all)—and whether or not that treatment should be continued under the current end-of-life circumstances.

More often than not, you will find that most palliative specialists will suggest stopping most medications. Pain medications are not, however, something to discontinue. Even if the patient, under hospice care at home, seems not to be in pain, we recommend continued use because pain meds have other benefits.

Many medications are administered on a schedule of one or two pills every six to eight hours. For an end-of-life situation, if the medication is designed for comfort and sense of well-being, and if the schedule is a little bit off kilter or out of whack, in the grand scheme of life, this really is not a big deal. Caregivers taking care of family members at home need to sleep too. If the overnight dose was missed, the world won't stop turning.

So the bottom line is that we need to be sensible—by which I mean, use the common sense that is not always common—focus on symptomatic and supportive interventions, and recognize that there needs to be flexibility in dealing with complex medical issues. The goal is comfort and quality of life.

15

How Can We Relieve Pain?

HE WAS ACTUALLY SUFFOCATING TO DEATH WHEN ADMITTED to our hospital late one night. His advanced lung cancer created pain and suffering, and the family was beside themselves, not knowing what to do and not wanting to see Grandpa so miserable. He was a farmer. A tough old man in his late seventies, he had worked every day of his life until cancer intervened.

Upon intake, those of us on hospital service that night saw a man not only in real pain but also clearly suffering psychologically and physiologically. With a small dose of morphine, intravenously administered, within approximately five minutes we saw a miraculous improvement. He was calm, he was able to breathe, and he even slept. He was able to spend his remaining days speaking comfortably with his family and without the dreaded fear of suffocation.

Without question, one of the most terrifying experiences of cancer patients and, in fact, patients with any chronic serious illness is the threat of living with and dying with pain.

The numbers are absolutely chilling. Approximately 40 percent of patients have severe pain toward the end of life. I'm talking about pain on the high end of the pain scale.

Clinicians often ask patients to rate their pain on a scale of 1 to 10, with 10 being the worst pain ever. Patients with pain (at least two-thirds of patients with cancer) will admit to a pain level of 8 or higher, and that's excruciating pain. Terrifying. Cruel and soul-shredding pain. Without the patient telling us about their pain, we cannot measure it with a scan or a blood test. (Children are given a scale of faces of pain to help them rank their pain levels.)

In general, we in the healthcare provider community have not been vigilant enough about this problem. Despite tremendous educational efforts to encourage providers to address patients' pain, about half of patients still receive inadequate pain management.

A number of years ago, the *Journal of the American Medical Association* published landmark research called the SUPPORT study. Very simplistically, a study was done of patients and families in intensive care units at major medical centers. In general, pain was a major issue for most patients, and there was inadequate communication between the family and the medical team in regard to the patient's wishes.

Therefore, an intensive educational program was launched on the use of medications for pain and how to have clear discussions with patients and families about pain management and symptom control. Guess what? The study clearly showed that despite intensive education, we continue to do a very poor job when it comes to alleviating suffering at the end of life.

So we on the palliative care team view ourselves as the advocate for the patient relative to pain management. One of the real advances in palliative medicine is definite evidence that the appropriate use of morphine and related drugs can dramatically enhance quality of life and sense of well-being for patients at the end of life. This remains the gold standard, and in the hands of credentialed professionals it is an absolute miracle drug.

Let us make an important distinction. Pain and suffering from the disease process is different from "total pain," which clearly has a spiritual, existential, or psychological component. All the morphine on the planet will not give a patient peace if their emotional, social, or spiritual issues are not recognized or acknowledged and resolved.

If a patient who is dying is receiving maximum pain medications and maximum interventions to decrease shortness of breath and treat insomnia and bowel/bladder problems, and that patient is still miserable, we need to think of an existential or a moral crisis. These "diseases of the soul" can only be addressed and healed by the attentive family and caregiver team who are open to possibilities.

I distinctly remember a gentleman dying of advanced pancreatic cancer. His pain was untouched by the highest doses we dared give him—to no avail. We later found out that he was approaching the anniversary of the tragic and sudden death of his son. Once we heard his story and acknowledged the source of his pain, we knew it was pain of the soul, which would not respond to morphine. We encouraged him to talk about the event with family and friends, which indeed helped ease his physical pain.

If we think back on our own personal experiences, when we are in pain, the focus of our world becomes very narrow. We are not thinking about family and engagements in the future; we are completely consumed with the toothache, the broken bone, or the kidney stone.

Now for a brief anatomy lesson. Throughout the spinal cord are "docking stations," or receptors, and morphine and related pain-relieving medications hook into these receptors and can clearly decrease pain.

We also need to understand that there are various types of pain that can only be clarified by a careful history and physical examination. It is also important for the clinician and the care team to have clear expectations and goals with patients and families. In almost all circumstances the pain can be improved even though it may not be completely eliminated.

An astonishing figure for patients and families to understand is that a competent medical professional can give 90 percent of cancer patients adequate pain relief so that their lives can be meaningful and focused and productive.

In general, we used to believe that a quickened pulse, sweating, and rapid breathing would be indications of pain, but this is not necessarily so. Patients should expect a careful physical examination of the skin, the soft tissue, the reflexes, and the painful area.

Under some circumstances, relatively simple laboratory studies and more complex investigations, such as the electromyogram (EMG), may be helpful, but in most circumstances, the history and physical examination will provide the necessary and important clues to pain management for palliative care purposes.

Pain is not the time for the patient to be a martyr or to "man up" or to endure. Pain can be relieved. Patients and caregivers need to tell the medical team about pain.

The Three-Step Approach to Treating Pain

Patients and families should have some basic understanding that there is a stepwise analysis in the use of medications to treat pain. Clinicians understand, in general, the use of the World Health Organization's analgesic ladder. This is a three-step approach, as follows:

1. For mild pain, patients would typically start with nonnarcotics, such as acetaminophen (Tylenol) or a nonsteroidal anti-inflammatory like ibuprofen (Advil).

   If this approach does not work, then we move to step 2.

2. This typically consists of an opioid medication, such as hydrocodone. Codeine used to be advised for this step, but the misery of constipation and nausea have made codeine much less appealing.

   If step 2 does not help the patient, we then move to step 3.

3. This typically would consist of opioid medications, such as morphine, oxycodone, or hydromorphone. It's important for

patients and families to understand that the pain medication must be taken on a fixed schedule, around the clock, rather than on a hit-or-miss schedule (also called PRN, or as needed). Patients should be carefully instructed, under most circumstances, to take the medication every four to six hours, as advised by the clinician, and to typically keep the medication with water at the bedside. Elderly patients can easily become confused during the night, and this is a setup for a fall if they have to get up to take their medications. The bathroom floor can be an unforgiving surface.

If patients are not doing well on one opioid, such as morphine, an alternative drug, such as hydrocodone, would be reasonable to try. There are tables and charts readily available to clinicians to switch from one dose to the next (these are called equianalgesic tables).

If feasible, keep a log of when the medication is taken. Nobody does this, in my experience. But we can properly prescribe if we know what was taken and when and how it worked or did not work. Write down dates, times, dosages, and pain levels.

And what about a combination? Let's discuss that. A commonly used term is coanalgesics. These are typically medications such as acetaminophen or nonsteroidal anti-inflammatory agents (as described in step 1) that can sometimes be added to a morphine program. In general, the acetaminophen dose should not be greater than 2.6 grams (2,600 mg) a day, and there is always concern that in the setting of excessive alcohol use, there could be substantial liver damage with acetaminophen. And then we're back to whether it would be a problem if Grandpa had a couple of beers while he was actively dying. Frankly, why would you deny him that pleasure? At end of life, liver damage is no longer an issue.

Some medications have specific risks and complications. For example, methadone, which was primarily used to treat addictive disorders, has a well-recognized place in the management of patients with cancer pain. However, an important warning: methadone can "hang around" for many days in the bloodstream, and the dose should only be increased under careful surveillance.

Methadone, along with such other medications as haloperidol, can cause life-threatening changes in the heart conduction system. Interestingly, grapefruit juice can also increase methadone levels to potentially dangerous concentrations (as this juice does with many other medications).

Under usual circumstances, a patient will take a specific dose of an opioid medication, such as morphine, about every four to six hours. This becomes very clumsy and uncomfortable and unwieldy for patients and families. After several days, usually, patients are more comfortable, and the rapidly acting opioid medication can then be converted into long-acting medicine, which is typically taken every twelve hours, around the clock. Most patients are given the liquid form for short-acting pain relief as drops under the tongue. The long-term version is swallowed as a tablet (not chewed because it releases too much at once).

What do we do if there is "breakthrough pain," which, for example, might occur a few hours after a dose of long-acting, twelve-hour pain medicine? If this does occur, patients are often then advised to take a rapidly acting dose of morphine, typically 5 to 10 milligrams, based on the patient's age and weight and other factors, so that there is a long-acting medication used in conjunction with the rapidly acting medication for breakthrough pain.

With modern medications, almost never is an intramuscular injection (a "shot") needed. These are painful, unpredictable, and in almost all circumstances, unnecessary.

Most cancer patients and families are aware of the "pain patch" (a transdermal [across the skin] technology about the size of a credit card). These medications can be helpful and are easily applied to the skin. Under usual circumstances, the patch is changed about every seventy-two hours. The patch should not be cut or manipulated. The pain patch takes twenty-four hours to kick in, so it's not used for an acute pain crisis. We place them on the chest wall or back. However, we have also learned that if the patient has a fever, this may cause a rapid absorption of the patch material, and patients may become confused.

Also, well-established medications can be placed under the tongue or between the cheek and the gum for patients who are not able to swallow.

Although usually not acceptable to most patients, there are rectal suppository forms of pain medications. This may be helpful for some end-of-life situations, but in general, this is not an ideal route of administration.

So, in summary, we can help patients to be relatively pain-free.

Controlling Side Effects of Pain Medications

Most patients and families are aware of the side effects of morphine and those sorts of pain medications, and we on the clinical side need to be proactive and preemptive in trying to avoid them.

Let me discuss some of the common side effects to watch for.

One of the most common miseries, which clearly erodes quality of life for many patients, is constipation. This is predictable. It will happen, and we need to be aggressive in treating it. Therefore, whenever hydrocodone or morphine is recommended for a patient, make sure the doctor also prescribes stool softeners.

Medications such as senna or bisacodyl are absolutely crucial to be taken, along with drinking a lot of water. Patients need to be asked about their bowel habits and patterns. If constipation seems to be occurring, an aggressive treatment plan must be put in place. As uncomfortable as it may be to ask your loved one if they have had a bowel movement—and when—these are vital pieces of information to report to the medical care team.

We also know that nausea and vomiting will be provoked in up to 40 percent of patients as a result of the use of some of these pain medications. Therefore, be especially attentive and, under some circumstances, talk with the care team about antinausea medicine at the same time the morphine is started.

Another issue that commonly arises involves confusion and cloudy thinking. For an elderly patient on multiple medications and with possible heart, kidney, or liver compromise, this is almost predictable. In general, the confusion and the fuzzy thinking are often a reflection of a combination of medicines, so the medical team must make a careful tabulation of what the patient is taking, and caregivers must be vigilant about Mom dosing herself with whatever she may have stashed in the medicine cabinet.

In fact, for caregivers at home, it is essential to remove any and all medicines, over-the-counter drugs, and vitamins and supplements that could be found in drawers and cabinets, on kitchen counters, and in purses. No need to complicate the medical management with unknown substances.

Usually, problems caused by taking many substances (called polypharmacy) are predictable, and they improve with careful attention to the medication schedule. These drug-drug interactions are why Grandma seems goofy.

There is another unusual complication that can be very disturbing, and we've already touched on it. It is called myoclonus—the sudden, rapid, and unpredictable jerking of arms and legs. This can occasionally awaken patients from sleep, and sometimes patients and families are concerned about a seizure or epilepsy. Usually, an explanation of this phenomenon can put to rest the fears of the patient and family. Just knowing about it will go a long way toward understanding what's going on.

Many patients and families are fearful of a decrease in breathing for a patient taking morphine. Almost never does this become life threatening. As patients become more acclimated to the medication, this situation usually improves, and there is no need for any type of antidote.

What about Addiction?

In the past, there was great angst in the medical community about loading up dying patients with morphine and fentanyl and other addictive pain meds in the form of pills and patches. It's not as if Grandma was ever going to rob a convenience store to get money to buy the drugs or go to rehab for addiction with meth users.

End of life is the time when the most powerful drugs in our arsenal are truly needed. You can carefully make the case if you are working with a physician who is reluctant to step up the pain-free game.

By definition, addiction to narcotics is a behavioral situation where patients have no control over drug usage; they compulsively crave the medication and will continue to use it despite obvious harm, such as automobile accidents or deterioration in business or personal relationships. Almost never—repeat after me—almost never does this occur among cancer patients.

But physical dependence is another matter. This means that if the pain medication is withdrawn, patients can develop symptoms like nausea, vomiting, diarrhea, tremulousness (shaking), and a general feeling of poor health. These are withdrawal symptoms, much like a patient going "cold turkey," by which we mean stopping the medication. This is why pain medications must be slowly tapered down if the patient has been on them for a period of time.

Now, there also is a phenomenon called pseudo addiction, which means that patients will seek the medication because of unrelieved pain. This typically happens when we on the provider side do not give enough dosage at a frequent-enough interval for pain relief (if pain recurs four to six hours after the last dose, the dose was not high enough, for example). When patients are given sensible doses at sensible intervals, there is no addictive concern.

There are obviously profound legal and social and ethical issues concerning the use of opioids such as morphine for pain medication. There is always the worry that if patients continue to take morphine, it will hasten death. Again, almost never is this an issue.

Now let's focus for a moment on the principle of double effect. This means, in specific terms, that morphine may be given for a patient's pain, and a predictable side effect of the morphine is that there may be a decrease in the patient's breathing rate, which might cause the patient to die.

The morphine was administered to treat the pain, not to accelerate the patient's death. The death was an inadvertent but completely anticipated side effect of treating the pain. This is an important principle that has been endorsed and supported by many religious thinkers and spiritual leaders and medical ethicists.

Legal and ethical circles discuss morphine as a secondary consequence. The primary consequence of the morphine is to decrease pain, not to accelerate the death of the patient. There are no compelling stories to demonstrate that the use of morphine or related opioids in any way accelerates the patient's death when used in an appropriate manner.

Intractable Pain

A complex problem, which is becoming more challenging, is assessing pain in the frail, demented individual. In general, dosages of all pain medications should be significantly *decreased* even up to 50 percent in the elderly, and nonverbal behaviors such as facial grimacing, irritability, and socialization may be tip-offs to a pain situation in someone who cannot speak for themselves or if their verbalizations don't seem rational.

In southeast Minnesota, we commonly deal with the stoic Northern European patient who has an incredibly high pain threshold, and we have to be persistent in trying to assess their actual level of discomfort. On the other hand, some cultures are far more demonstrative and vocal in their description of pain, and these factors must clearly be taken into account in managing a pain situation.

Sometimes, however, the best of narcotic medicines simply do not work or stop working. Intractable pain is what we call it. And this type of pain is not only brutal on the patient, it's excruciating for the family at the bedside.

Technical interventions such as spinal cord pumps and nerve blocks can be considered, without doubt, for patients with an expected survival of approximately two to three months. This discussion would take place with a pain specialist, typically an anesthesiologist.

These devices can be sometimes clumsy for families and patients to handle, but no patient should be denied the input of that type of technology, especially if the survival is expected to be longer than three months.

Steroids

One of the most underutilized and important medications for patients with serious illness, especially at the end of life, are corticosteroids or steroids. These medications are typically called prednisone or Decadron or dexamethasone. These drugs not only have a role to play in attacking the cancer pain, but often can increase appetite, mood, and sense of well-being. In some circumstances, these medications can decrease the swelling around tumors and provide the patient with relief.

Over a long period of time, there are side effects of these medications, such as a "moon face," as well as fungal infections of the mouth, diabetes, and weight gain. However, the use of the judicious, sensible dose in the advanced cancer patient can provide striking benefits.

Antidepressants

We also have learned that antidepressants may have an important role to play in patients with pain. If depression seems to be exacerbating or worsening a pain situation, a rapidly acting antidepressant would be very important. However, as I previously mentioned, the time for the antidepressant to kick in may be four to six weeks. In this situation, a medication such as methylphenidate or Ritalin would be helpful, since a conservative dose can act rapidly and increase mood and sense of well-being within several days.

Alternative Medicine

Many patients and families also raise the issue of alternative and complementary therapies when dealing with pain. Without doubt, mind-body approaches and the use of guided imagery, psychological interventions, massage therapy, music, and acupuncture are reasonable interventions. A meditation app on an iPhone or a visualization CD played through earbuds can be comforting to both the patient and the family caregiver.

An often underutilized professional group in dealing with the patient in pain is the physical therapist. Gentle stretching exercises and the use of free weights and resistance bands are often helpful.

So what have I learned from patients in dealing with pain? An important lesson is that pain dramatically deteriorates quality of life and erodes the personality and the demeanor of the patient, who may become demanding, unreasonable, and even irrational. You would too if you had vomiting and nausea, were not sleeping, and saw no light at the end of the tunnel.

In the palliative world, I have seen patients aggressively treated with morphine and steroids for their pain, with an aggressive bowel prep to relieve constipation, with meds to aid in sleeping, and within a day or two, there has been a miraculous transformation in the patient. We of course did not treat or cure the life-ending illness, but we made the patient's remaining time much more pain-free and comfortable.

16

How Do We Control Other Symptoms?

PAIN ISN'T THE ONLY SYMPTOM THE CARE TEAM NEEDS TO address, but it's the most difficult and the most debilitating. Other symptoms cause misery for patients and families, and these are called nonpain symptoms. Of course, family caregivers need to be vigilant and report symptoms to the medical care team or call the hospice nurse for guidance.

Let's address the symptoms to watch for.

Fear of Suffocation, Shortness of Breath

One of the greatest fears of patients is that of suffocation or drowning, especially for individuals with cancers of the lung and the head and neck area. The clinical term for this fear is dyspnea, and it's one of the symptoms that clearly worsens as death approaches.

Much like pain, dyspnea is the discomfort reported by the patient. It cannot be measured by an oxygen monitor or blood test; so if the patient says, "I am short of breath," we the care providers, and the family, must listen to that patient.

We have come a long way in understanding why patients are short of breath, and one of the mainstays of treatment is that of a very careful dose of morphine. As mentioned, a few milligrams intravenously or a similarly low dose of liquid placed under the tongue (sublingual) or inside the cheek can be of enormous value in decreasing that suffering.

A cornerstone of medical management is to determine why the patient is short of breath. If there is fluid in the lung, occasionally that can be tapped off. If there is evidence of pneumonia or anemia, there are interventions to help relieve those issues as well.

I'll repeat an image and insight shared earlier: We've all seen the dog with his face draped outside the car window taking in the breeze. Interestingly, we now know that there are nerve endings in the facial area, and when air is blown over these areas as with a fan, there can be a dramatic decrease in shortness of breath. Putting a small fan or cool-mist humidifier to blow across the bed of the patient is obviously a low-risk intervention and certainly should be considered.

The issue always arises about supplemental oxygen, typically through a mask or nasal prongs. The mask becomes disabling in that patients cannot speak comfortably, and the nasal prongs are also uncomfortable, and nobody ever gets them situated properly. They just seem to slide around and away from the nostrils.

A usual approach is to measure the patient's blood oxygen level with that little clip-on device on a finger, and if oxygen levels are below a certain number, then supplemental oxygen may be of value. However, in many patients, there does not seem to be a correlation between the feeling of dyspnea and suffocation and what the oxygen level is. So the bottom line is clear: listen to the patient.

If a patient is short of breath, a vicious cycle ensues where that patient becomes anxious and that induces more breathlessness. Medications called benzodiazepines (Xanax or Valium, for example) can decrease anxiety and be an important addition to a more traditional morphine program.

Likewise, patients with shortness of breath often have congestion from pooled secretions. A dose of a diuretic/water medicine called Lasix (furosemide) can be helpful in keeping patients at home and out of the hospital. There are also medications by mouth and by vein, such as glycopyrrolate, which are sometimes considered to be helpful in decreasing the accumulations of secretions and the discomfort that follows. Occasionally, a patch of scopolamine behind the ear may be of great help.

Inability to Swallow, Fear of Choking

Another misery for patients is difficulty in swallowing (called dysphagia). This leads the patient to worry about choking. The reason for this suffering might be something as simple as poorly fitting dentures or other dental problems, magnified by stress, tension, and anxiety. A simple solution would be to remove the dentures, of course, and see if that relieves the problem.

But there may be far more ominous reasons for dysphagia, such as neurologic diseases, including ALS (Lou Gehrig's disease).

It is important for the palliative care team to embark upon a thorough assessment to help target the therapy. Dryness of the mouth caused by radiation or medications or a fungal infection is very treatable.

Frozen ice chips and Popsicles and attention to oral hygiene, as simple as they sound, can sometimes make a world of difference in addressing this issue.

Lack of Appetite, Weight Loss

Food and meals are profoundly symbolic and are associated with almost every significant human interaction. The wedding, the baptism, the confirmation, the bar mitzvah—even annual events like birthdays and anniversaries—are typically associated with a meal. So when patients are not able to eat on a regular basis and lose weight, this opens up a whole portfolio of anguish, especially on the part of the family. The primary caregiver often feels frustrated and underappreciated, especially if the caregiver brings all the patient's favorite foods to the bedside—to no avail.

However, we now recognize that for many patients the cause of the illness produces chemicals or peptides or hormones or some substance that clearly interferes with appetite and the processing of food. In many circumstances, this difficulty cannot be overridden by forcing the patient to eat. However, there are some well-recognized and sometimes not always considered interventions.

If patients are nauseated and simply have no desire to eat, a medication such as metoclopramide may increase the action of the stomach and the intestinal tract.

Peer review trials of a medication called megestrol acetate clearly show that it increases weight and appetite, but not necessarily lean muscle mass. The medication can be given in tablet or liquid form and plays a really important role in enhancing weight gain in the patient, with relatively few side effects (blood clots are a concern but are rare).

An issue that almost always arises is the role of providing high-calorie nutrition in patients with advanced disease. It seems intuitive that if we provide the patient with artificial hydration and nutrition, they will be better able to withstand chemotherapy and may have a better survival, but this is not always the case. On occasion, these interventions may worsen the patient's outcome because of wild swings in body chemistry provoking diarrhea and the risk of infection.

I'm talking here about a feeding tube, and I have discussed how it works elsewhere in this book. The decision to start (and when to stop) is huge.

Although the medical literature is not consistent in this area, for some patients with ALS, esophageal or obstructive cancers, or an acute stroke, artificial nutrition should be carefully considered by the family and the patient so that there is a clear understanding of expectations and an acknowledgment that these interventions sometimes hasten the patient's death and increase rates of complications.

There's often no need to bake Grandma's favorite strudel or bring a cup of her favorite soup to the bedside. Bottom line is that family members are often comforted when a member of the medical team explains the patient's lack of eating this way: Grandma is not dying because she isn't eating. She's not eating because she is dying.

A comfort measure for the person who is not eating or drinking is to keep ice chips nearby, sponge the mouth and lips, and apply lip balm or petroleum jelly to the lips.

Incontinence

Toileting is always an issue for someone confined to bed or with limited mobility. A bedside commode can often be brought in from a home health supplier. The person may wear incontinence pads or Depends-type underwear. For some patients a catheter may be used.

Inability to Speak

A patient on a ventilator cannot speak. Sometimes hand gestures are used, but often the patient's hands are secured so they cannot pull out the vent either on purpose or by accident. Even for someone in a twilight sleep, which is often protocol when on a vent (that is, they are lightly sedated), the person can hear you but not be able to respond coherently.

Sit beside them, hold their hand, and gently talk and reassure them where they are and what you wish to say, understanding that they cannot respond except with a hand squeeze. Patients not on a ventilator but not speaking may respond to hand holding.

Fatigue

This is beyond simply being tired, beyond the kind of tired an afternoon nap cures. I'm talking about profound fatigue—an overwhelming exhaustion that utterly drains and depletes—you can't really describe.

This is almost a given for most cancer patients at the end of life, and there are many explanations: anemia, malnutrition, depression, pain, or simply being in bed.

We know from many studies that for every day in bed, it might require one or two days of activity for that patient to regain a previous level of fitness. Obviously, many patients with advanced disease will no longer leave their beds, but early in the course of a patient's illness there should be some careful thought to the role of the physical therapist.

As mentioned, a gentle program of stretching and resistance work with bands or free weights can often provide a tremendous stimulus to increase the appetite and the patient's sense of well-being. It's unclear if long-lasting benefits may derive from these programs, but certainly PT helps the patient participate in their care.

Nausea and Vomiting

Among the most disheartening and disabling symptoms verbalized by patients are nausea and vomiting. If we just think about our own personal experiences, even a tinge of nausea can be profoundly debilitating, and I see it with at least two-thirds of cancer patients.

There are multiple reasons for nausea and vomiting, and a careful history and physical examination, in conjunction with appropriate imaging interventions and blood studies, are absolutely crucial. As a rule of thumb, up to 80 percent of patients with nausea can be improved when there is a careful history, physical examination, and the appropriate use of medications.

The three areas that really need to be investigated are the brain and the intestinal tract, as well an acknowledgment that the patient's medications (for example, chemotherapy) may play a major role in nausea.

I mention the brain because increased pressure in the brain, typically from a brain tumor, can show up as nausea or vomiting. In some patients, we routinely obtain an MRI of the head and surprisingly find a large brain tumor that explains the nausea, with no other symptoms being present.

I'm reminded of a situation several years ago where a patient became nauseated as she drove through a small town on her way to receive chemotherapy. The name of the town was Thomasville, and the chemotherapy nurse had the first name of Thomas; so, as the patient saw the sign indicating the name of the town, she was triggered with nausea and vomiting. We cannot discount the emotional issues.

A whole array of medications can be administered orally, rectally, or subcutaneously by injection, and all cancer physicians are familiar with these programs. But these measures can only be used if, indeed, the patient verbalizes how disabling the nausea is.

Bowel Obstruction

A disastrous complication of intra-abdominal cancer is the dreaded bowel obstruction. Historically, these patients had a nasogastric tube placed through their nose and down into the intestines to suck out the fluid, or some required surgery from which the recovery was long and painful. Many patients never returned to their previous level of comfort.

However, with the appropriate use of multiple medications there has been a resurgence of interest in medications to alleviate a bowel blockage without the use of an uncomfortable tube or surgery. There are standard protocols involving morphine and related medications, other medicines to decrease the secretions in the intestine, and medications to control the muscular contraction of the bowel wall.

We have finally reached a point in history where patients can be spared the discomfort of surgery. In some circumstances, there can be a meaningful relief of the bowel blockage without surgery.

Delirium, Confusion

A profoundly disabling observation, especially among family members, is delirium, which is defined as the fluctuating and/ or altered level of consciousness. Patients may be hyperactive with agitation, anxiety, and constant movement, or they may have a hypoactive variety, which is sleepiness, indifference, and withdrawn behavior. Patients are inattentive. They can be profoundly disruptive and disorganized.

One of the first assessments is a careful evaluation of the patient's medications, especially any new drugs. It is also essential to recognize that imbalances in body minerals, as well as disturbances in liver or kidney function, can have a dramatic impact on the cause of delirium.

Psychotropic medications, such as haloperidol, risperidone, olanzapine, and lorazepam, may be prescribed. But a profound word of caution here. At a recent board review course sponsored by the American Academy of Hospice and Palliative Medicine, the experts acknowledged that if 100 patients with delirium are treated with these kinds of medications, approximately 7 to 10 will get better; approximately 7 to 10 may well die from the risks of the medication; and the rest of the patients remain basically the same.

So, as is usually the case in medicine, there needs to be a thoughtful discussion with the medical care team regarding the pros, cons, risks, and potential benefits.

On the other hand, flying in the face of common sense, dehydration may be the culprit and should be assessed. Dehydration is profoundly debilitating. Many patients simply feel better once they are hydrated rather than being in a dehydrated state. Hydration is achieved through IV fluids if the patient cannot drink at least 60 ounces of water each day. This is a short-term, often onetime, IV treatment and not administered at the very end of life or over the long term.

Lack of Sleep

On an equally important note, we cannot ignore for a moment the erosion of quality of life from lack of sleep. This can have a devastating impact on both patients and families. If patients are not sleeping, a careful review of the medication schedule is absolutely crucial. For example, steroid medications and other medicines when taken late in the day or early in the evening will dramatically interfere with sleep, and the next day becomes a nightmare.

In general, sleeping medications only have a temporary impact on most patients, but for the advanced cancer patient the use of these agents—and a switch to alternative agents if the first medicine is not effective—is reasonable.

At the end of someone's life, families look back and may not remember the skilled surgeon or the radiologist, but they certainly remember the nurse who provided a warm blanket or the physical therapist who performed a daily foot massage. The family member who turned down the lights, played soothing music, and just sat by the bedside. The neighbor who brought over a pan of lasagna or a batch of lemon bars. The hospice nurse who helped with a sponge bath. The grandchild who stood by the bedside and with all the innocence of childhood said, "Grandma, I love you."

17

How Do Doctors Manage the Diseases of Death?

ONCE SOMEONE HAS DIED, WE ON THE MEDICAL TEAM WILL provide information for the death certificate. Cause of death is one of the items we fill in. Of course, heart disease is the leading cause of death, followed closely by cancer. Among the top causes are COPD/emphysema (largely caused by smoking), stroke, dementia, and diabetes.

But it's not unusual to find causes of death that are more obscure. These might include hidden infections, or blood clots in the legs, which can often spread into the lungs and cause death. What actually causes death may not be the disease process itself but complications from a disease.

At the bedside, the cause of death is less important to those of us on the palliative team than caring for the patient's symptoms and making them comfortable and pain-free. These diseases of death discussed in this chapter pose their own challenges. Let me address some of them.

Congestive Heart Failure

With the tremendous advances in the medical management of patients with heart disease, patients are living far longer than ever. Heart failure is typically defined by the New York Heart Association Classification System of 1 through 4, where 1 involves symptoms of fatigue, shortness of breath, or rapid pulse only with more than ordinary activity, progressing to stage 4 with symptoms at rest. This condition becomes even more complicated, since approximately 80 percent of patients who are hospitalized with heart failure are sixty-five years of age or older.

Patients not only develop shortness of breath and a decreased exercise capability (a flight of stairs, for example, would be daunting) but also have major cognitive impairment in total and memory recall, compared with a general population. Interestingly, it is not well acknowledged that studies now show that up to 40 percent of patients have severe pain with heart failure.

Until several years ago, patients who died of heart disease typically died from an electrical failure in the heart or an irregularity in the heart rhythm or blocked blood vessels. However, today, we see chronic heart failure. Patients suffer from massively swollen legs, for example. They are short of breath and have profoundly distressing total body aching. That's real pain, and it's why we treat heart patients for pain.

In some medical settings, it is now customary for the palliative care team to be intimately involved with the management of patients with congestive heart failure. Their symptoms are complicated and clearly decrease quality of life—shortness of breath is a major issue, so medications to treat anxiety, a low-dose benzodiazepine like Ativan (lorazepam), can be especially helpful.

As the clinical disease trajectory unfolds, these patients will continue to retain fluid and often have shortness of breath as a major issue. Very conservative doses of morphine can be of tremendous value, and a dose under the tongue of haloperidol can often modify the anxiety of these patients.

Medical management has become especially complicated with the evolution of technology called the left ventricular assist device (LVAD), as previously mentioned. After one year of having this mechanical pumping device in place, 85 to 90 percent of patients are still alive with a better quality of life than before the device was inserted.

Nevertheless, these complex technical interventions require the tremendous support of engaged family members who are physically fit and emotionally stable enough to deal with the complications of these devices.

Because of the role of technology, the withdrawing of life-prolonging therapies becomes a challenging and often dramatic discussion with patients and families. The advance care planning is especially complicated because of the use of the defibrillator, which can be implanted under the skin. Talk with your medical care team about the do not resuscitate (DNR) orders and whether or not to deactivate these devices.

Usually, these discussions don't take place at all, but I think they are absolutely important for patient empowerment. These implanted defibrillators may continue to fire and shock the patient toward the end of life, and this can be profoundly disabling. Families need to understand that as the device continues to fire, it will not save the patient's life but certainly increase the suffering.

So, in the light of day and during a quiet moment, there really needs to be a thoughtful discussion about how this device can be deactivated and what the patient's wishes are in this regard. There are well-established legal and moral guidelines indicating that under some circumstances when the LVAD is not meeting the goals of the patient, it is appropriate to deactivate it with a credit card–type device (not surgery).

I acknowledge that these are very painful discussions and decisions and need to be made with a thoughtful review by the patient, the family, the spiritual support community, as well as the clinicians caring for the patient.

When these devices are deactivated, most patients die within approximately twenty minutes, so the family needs to be aware of this timeline. Typically, the palliative care team has been engaged with the end-stage cardiac patient toward the end of life. But now there is an increasing awareness about the value of this service, and the palliative care team is often invited to engage the patient early in the clinical course so that our relationship can be forged. The difficulties with the late-stage referral are that the average stay for some cardiac patients at a hospice program is only ten days. This is hardly enough time for the family to engage the work of grieving and to address the needs of the patient.

Dementia

Every several weeks in the media we read about a celebrity or athlete or prominent personality struggling with dementia. Most of us know someone whose quality of life is unraveling from this disastrous situation. Data show that someone is diagnosed with Alzheimer's dementia every seventy-one seconds.

The impact on our communities and on the healthcare system is absolutely overwhelming. We now recognize that there are several types of dementia, with Alzheimer's disease accounting for approximately one-third of dementia. Other types of dementia are caused by strokes and blood vessel disorders or relatively unusual neurologic disorders, such as Lewy body dementia.

The actual type of dementia is less important than its management. And we can only confirm the type of dementia during an autopsy when pathologists look at the brain itself.

A quick glance at our changing American society underscores that age is the greatest risk factor for dementia. About 50 percent of people over age eighty-five will have some evidence of dementia—which, over the next several decades, means a number equivalent to the current population of New York City.

Dementia can be a lingering illness with a survival of about five to eight years after diagnosis, and the treatment options are medical, behavioral, environmental, and psychological.

A number of FDA-approved medications certainly can be considered in some of these patients. Yet only about 15 to 20 percent of patients get some benefit from such medications as donepezil or Aricept (but the medication causes nausea, vomiting, and diarrhea, which are not symptoms an older person needs). There does seem to be some improvement, or at least stabilization, in the symptoms of dementia in these patients, and there may be a delay in nursing home placement. But that's it. No cure. Nothing promising in the drug pipeline either.

It was once thought that dementia would not actually be a cause of death—that someone would die *with* the disease—but that is not correct. Dementia causes death by starvation and infection.

One of the real challenges in dealing with dementia patients involves the assessment of hospice eligibility. Because of the disease's variable and unpredictable clinical course, guidelines have been challenging. But most hospice organizations follow some guidelines to consider hospice eligibility.

For example, if patients cannot walk, dress, or bathe without assistance, are incontinent, and cannot speak more than six different intelligible words per day, they may be hospice candidates. The assessment of the foregoing pertinent criteria is called the FAST score (Functional Assessment Staging Test) and is well known to the palliative care community. I invite you to perform a Google search to see the levels of abilities ranked. There are also other factors to be considered, such as weight loss and certain laboratory studies. If the criteria are not met, patients are not eligible for hospice placement, even though they might require intensive medical care and supervision.

We cannot ignore symptom management in these patients, even though they may not be able to tell us they have pain. Up to 80 percent of dementia patients in long-term care facilities have a pain situation. If they can't talk to us, we must look for nonverbal clues as to pain, such as behavioral changes, facial expressions, and grimacing.

An incredibly disabling and frightening observation is agitation, which can occur in up to half of patients struggling with dementia. There are multiple causes for agitation, such as pain and psychological issues, being in an unfamiliar environment, medications, and also dementia itself. Agitation is particularly frightening and upsetting for family members to witness.

Mealtimes can be especially challenging, since some patients simply don't recognize utensils, and the commotion and the energy of the dining area can be overwhelming. Some seem to stop eating. I have seen family members quietly feeding their loved ones in their rooms in a nursing facility, which raises the agonizing question about whether we continue nutrition in any form in dementia patients.

As dementia progresses, families are confronted with profound ethical issues. One of these is the use of the feeding tube, typically placed through the abdominal wall into the stomach. We've already discussed feeding tubes. In terms of our discussion in regard to dementia, let me outline the key issues. The mortality is high from these procedures, for practical reasons, and is often associated with aspiration pneumonia where secretions pool in the lungs and create an infectious, inflammatory component. Antibiotics are not consistently effective in treating these infections.

We now have evidence that the tube feedings do not enhance quality of life or well-being and do not promote wound healing in demented patients. This requires an in-depth family discussion, since the knee-jerk reflex in many circumstances is to insert the tube.

Families and the primary caregiver can often feel an overwhelming sense of futility. These types of cases are often the most difficult for everyone, which is why a thoughtful discussion (or, perhaps, several) with the doctor is required. The feeding tube is not appropriate. Nor is spoon-feeding the far-advanced patient. Why? Because such feedings prolong the dying process (in the case of cancer, feedings effectively feed the tumor).

We recommend that Dad be taken home to die in peace and dignity with his family rather than under the glare of the ICU monitors, or made comfortable in a nursing home or hospice bed with familiar items and family members present.

These are among the most painful decisions a family will ever make. Looking back, most are grateful to have received and followed the wise advice of the palliative team and reassured in knowing their loved one was made comfortable in a final passing.

Chronic Obstructive Pulmonary Disease (COPD)

COPD, more commonly referred to as emphysema, has become a global pandemic primarily fueled by smoking. Much like with dementia, it is difficult to accurately predict mortality or the death rate for patients with advanced COPD.

We know, for example, that breathing studies in conjunction with a limited ability to walk, complicated by depression and social isolation and recurrent hospitalization, predict an increased risk of dying within twelve months of diagnosis. However, in any one patient, it is of course difficult to bring to the bedside a specific timetable of survival.

These patients may be on oxygen, taking bronchodilators and medications called long-acting anticholinergics. Some may be getting steroids, although the long-term benefit is controversial. Some may be using inhalers.

The palliative care community can play a major role in the management of these patients, especially as their needs escalate toward the end of life. Without question, there needs to be a clear acknowledgment of anxiety and depression as shortness of breath worsens. Patients fear suffocating, as described earlier in this chapter.

We know that depression should be acknowledged and treated under appropriate circumstances, since this disorder can be an independent predictor of death in patients with advanced COPD. Because of the unpredictable clinical course of COPD and the revolving door of emergency room and hospital admissions, a timely family conference at some point is absolutely crucial to decrease delays in end-of-life decision-making.

An important question is whether or not the patient would want intubation or mechanical ventilation, while acknowledging that it might not be possible to remove the breathing device and the patient would be sustained on a respirator for an indefinite period of time. It's at this point that the hospice community can provide an important intervention, since the criteria for hospice admission for these patients would assess progressive shortness of breath, even at rest, and low oxygen levels and heart failure. We also look for weight loss.

These sorts of criteria would really warrant an in-depth discussion with the medical care team as to the patient's wishes and decisions should the patient begin to deteriorate.

As this chapter closes, let me underscore that I have addressed the cancer issues throughout because that is my specialty, so I will not spend time here on managing these end-of-life concerns. Suffice it to say, the spiritual issues of patients with any of these chronic diseases that most assuredly will cause death can often be profound. It is also critical to acknowledge and address the spiritual needs of the family members, most especially the primary family caregiver(s).

The crucial issue is quality of life and quality of death and the costs of supportive interventions, such as feeding tubes, artificial hearts, kidney dialysis, respirators, and other advanced technologies and devices. Costs are not measured in terms of money or insurance. These interventions do not cure, and their use exacts a profound spiritual cost on those left behind.

18

What Does "Do Not Resuscitate" (DNR) Really Mean?

"DOCTOR, THE PATIENT IS CODING."

"Call a code blue. Get me a crash cart," says the extremely handsome doctor rushing into the patient's room.

"Clear," he calls out as he applies electronic paddles to the chest, and the cardio monitor starts beeping.

"He's back."

Exciting, isn't it? Real? Nah. TV doctor.

In real life, the elderly nursing home patient is found unconscious and rushed in an ambulance with a paramedic perched over the patient on the gurney giving CPR compressions, breaking feeble ribs, as the ambulance speeds to the emergency room where the heart is shocked and the patient is placed on a respirator and kidney machines and has a dreadful end-of-life experience—if they survive the experience at all.

How can these sorts of nightmares be minimized?

Only a minuscule percentage of patients who are resuscitated leave the hospital, and only a small percentage return to their previous level of functioning. So, even if Uncle Harry is resuscitated, the probability of an unfortunate outcome is astonishingly high.

This stark reality has led to the evolution of "physicians' orders for life-sustaining treatments" or the POLST document (a shorter version of the patient's advance directive). This is a life-enhancing document in which patients clearly spell out what they want when it comes to cardiopulmonary resuscitation: DNR with "comfort measures" or CPR and "full treatment." This document is kept with the patient, much like we keep our driver's license with us, and really puts the patient at the center of these difficult decision-making processes. Assisted living and nursing homes have these orders handy (sometimes on the back of the person's door).

But the paramedics at your door don't stop to ask about a document. If someone calls 911, the emergency responders do just that—respond to the emergency.

For our purposes here, let me address just the resuscitate part. To resuscitate means that the patient would be intubated. In other words, placed on a breathing machine, and the heart would be shocked in an attempt to restore normal rhythm. You've seen it on TV a million times.

Without a document from you or your healthcare surrogate/decision-maker, those of us in medical healthcare will pull out all stops to prevent you from dying. We will provide the medications needed to restart your heart, and we will provide the mechanical aspects of putting a tube into your throat to breathe for you.

Before we go further, please understand that emergency measures are appropriate for most people in tragic accidents and other dire situations, but I am discussing patients at the end of their lives who are gravely ill. At the end of life, emergency measures are not actions you want. Nature is taking its course, and no matter what an alarmed family member says, if you "code"—in other words, your heart and ability to breathe are not working—we on the medical team are committed to restoring those functions. This is a full court press.

Without emergency medical measures, you will likely die peacefully, without a paramedic compressing your chest, breaking your ribs, and without paddles shocking you—a natural death.

To me, that seems reasonable.

Consider this: For someone in an end-of-life situation, such as heart disease or advanced cancer, there is little justification for resuscitation. If the patient is revived, they will only die from the primary condition anyway. This is a far different situation from someone injured in a car accident, unconscious, trapped in the vehicle or lying in the street, who is resuscitated and whisked away to a hospital by paramedics.

Later in this book, I discuss the advance directive—a document that spells out your wishes if you are in a medical crisis. I list websites where you can download the document and fill it out. (See chapters 21 and 22 for more details on the advance directive.)

If you choose, the directive known as DNR, or do not resuscitate, is indicated on your medical record in the hospital; on your files in nursing homes, sometimes on the doors; behind the door of an apartment or residence; in a pocket or folder; or on a bracelet.

My coauthor was alarmed to see several shelves of black binders in the nursing office at her mother's assisted living facility. Clearly marked on most of the three-inch spines were yellow letters spelling out D-N-R.

"Why aren't all the patients DNR?" she asked, only to be informed that the handful of residents without the DNR stickers still wanted every measure taken to revive them. They would get the paramedic compressing their chest and a fast ride to the hospital, where they would—well, remember, we doctors aren't God, so we don't absolutely know the outcome. Most likely, though, those patients would not return to assisted living.

Choosing the DNR directive is a decision that patients are asked to make. And if they can't, their healthcare surrogate is asked to make it, in advance. Not at the moment of code. Without a healthcare surrogate, family members are asked. Imagine the chaos at the bedside if Grandpa codes, nothing is in place, and the family is not in agreement. At that point, the charmingly handsome doctor—me, in this instance—calls for the crash cart and paddles.

In the end-stage patient, resuscitation is clearly not called for. Until the late 1980s, it was the medical staff who determined who would be resuscitated. There has been a tremendous shift in this position, and now patients can ask for resuscitation even though the probability of benefit is limited.

We know from studies in the medical journals that no more than 18 percent, or one patient in six, following resuscitation would be dismissed from the hospital, and a proportion of those patients have significant brain damage because of the lack of blood flow to the brain.

When individuals are admitted to a hospital, there are often clumsy discussions about resuscitation, typically with the stressed-out, exhausted patient at night. The usual inquiry goes something like this. The nurse asks, "Okay, if your heart stops, do you want us to shock it back? Do you want us to do CPR?"

The logical and informed patient would say, "Yes, of course," but this often belies the reality of the situation. If a patient is focusing on comfort measures and palliative care, to resuscitate that patient is inconsistent with that patient's wish. So there needs to be a thoughtful discussion that CPR is not consistent with the patient's stated wish, and then we can plan accordingly. The bottom line is this: studies show that few patients at the end of life who are resuscitated in a hospital setting ever leave the hospital in a relatively normal state.

19

How Do We Make Sense of Deathbed Confessions?

"HEY, DOC, AREN'T YOU HEADED HOME?" A PATIENT ASKED ME one evening as I was making final rounds during my weekly rotation on what we call hospital service. I was slotted in as the attending several weeks a year, and with a top-notch nursing team and residents and fellows, we covered about forty patients at any given time, all at the end of their lives.

His nightlight was on. His skeletal head and neck sank deeply into a nest of pillows. This diminutive figure, a ninety-year-old man from a small town in Missouri who had been admitted to the hospital with advanced lung cancer wanted to talk. I wanted to listen.

He began the story of his service in World War II. "You know I was with the engineers on those islands in the Pacific. Our battalion built hangars and water systems and sewers on those little spits of land. I loved it. 'Course, I was just out of high school when the war started. We all signed up, you know."

Between coughing spells, he told me about how he gained skills in home construction. He envisioned how cities would have housing booms once "that damned war" was over. He foresaw the baby boomers. And there he was, positioned to carve out an incredibly prosperous career once he returned to the States.

"But my dad needed me. No guys were left to work there, and the women hated it. So he wanted me back there running the store with him. I had no choice," he told me with regret, describing his dad's hardware store in the small Missouri town.

"So no bridges or roads or water treatment plants for you?"
I asked.

"No, closest I got was selling hammers and screws. I was never
happy working there." He blamed his unhappiness on several
failed relationships over the years. "Too late now to cry about
that," he said. But the sadness of those years was reflected on
his face as he looked away. I knew he was deep in thought, processing what days he had left, and I quietly slipped out the door.

I never knew if he shared that regret with his children and
grandchildren. But I hear many deathbed confessions and regrets.

Having been touched by about 40,000 encounters with the
terminally ill and having maintained a clinical curiosity, for me,
it is fascinating to listen to the stories of patients at the end of life.
When death is near, when the eleventh-hour reprieve has been
rejected by the governor, there really is no need for dishonesty.

My white coat becomes almost a priestly collar, the hospital
room a confessional, and that doctor/patient interaction an
opportunity to set the record straight.

Here are some of the themes I hear at the bedside confessional: missing opportunities, both personally and professionally;
not mending fences; wasting talents; staying with an abusive
partner; working hard for the gold watch and realizing too late
that there was more to life; squandering chances; giving in to
worry, fear, and dread; remaining in unfulfilling relationships;
having estranged children or spouses; not speaking to a parent
or sibling because of some long-forgotten squabble; giving up
children for adoption; questioning the afterlife (especially for
members of the clergy); regretting never-recouped losses (of
money or anything else); feeling unvalidated because of same-sex
relationships never brought out of the closet and/or alternative
lifestyles never acknowledged; feeling overwhelmed by family
secrets, secret affairs, or any intimate secrets never revealed.

These themes represent life's what-ifs.

A number of patients were despondent that they didn't have
the courage to have pushed the envelope with their investments

or their business activities: The shopping center that wasn't built. The library that wasn't finished. The political office that was never reached. All these can weigh heavily on the souls of individuals at the end of life. Interestingly, their angst was not so much about money or the trappings of success, but, rather, that they would die thinking they would leave no legacy and soon be forgotten.

Consider Whittier's quote: "Of all sad words of tongue or pen, the saddest are these, 'It might have been.'" In other words, *I'll never know how good I could have been.* Many were regretful that they hadn't trained hard enough. They hadn't studied hard enough, they hadn't practiced enough, and they were surpassed on the corporate or professional treadmill by someone of lesser skill but greater determination.

I hear regrets about missing a special birthday party, a hockey tournament, a child's play, that meal with friends and family, and opportunities to be with family and friends—all because of now-meaningless business meetings, business travel, or work deadlines.

There also were regrets of not having reached out to that colleague, friend, or neighbor during a difficult divorce, the death of a child, or some financial setback. A very close colleague whom I cared for at the end of life was regretful that she never picked up that phone, never wrote that note, never shook the hand of another colleague who was languishing under the crushing burden and the glare of publicity of a lawsuit that had absolutely no merit whatsoever.

So, what I heard, and what I continue to hear, are regrets about missed opportunities of not connecting with friends and family, not providing that hug or a handshake. Somehow, these actions are what most enrich the fabric of our lives. It was not about stuff money can buy; rather, their confessions were attempts to heal the wounds of our fellow travelers on the journey of life.

I also often heard about having to march to the beat of someone else's drummer. The regret of having felt like a puppet when someone else was pulling the strings. A bad boss. An abusive spouse. A demanding parent. A controlling sibling.

Another phenomenon that was equally common and always disturbing is the individual who just about reached the pinnacle of their career or profession but fell short, only to blame the coach, the manager, the agent, the boss, the tenure committee, or whichever political party was in the White House. There was no sense of personal responsibility. There was no asking the question, "Okay, this or that happened. What role did I play in this mess?"

Nevertheless, at the eleventh hour, most of these individuals shared with me that when they were honest with themselves, they did realize that they were not as focused, they were not as fanatical about success, they became sloppy in their preparation. These were the reasons for their failure—it was not someone else's fault, and it was not because of some cosmic misalignment of the stars. It was simply because they didn't work hard enough or failed to remain focused on the task at hand.

At the bedside, in my role as medical professional, I am safe. I am anonymous, and patients feel a real need to unburden themselves to another human being regarding their setbacks and failures. I do not judge. I listen.

How to Start the Bedside Conversation

The vigil at the bedside of someone dying is a time of great drama. Emotions unravel. Past histories can become painful or comforting. Distant relatives may suddenly appear. And in most circumstances, legal and financial issues are never completely resolved. So what can family members do during this time of great potential peace and great potential peril?

There is overwhelming evidence for the "power of presence." This means just showing up, without the need to say anything— even if you feel compelled to say something. Each of us has some genetic traits for compassion, and there is a fundamental human tendency to do something, even if that something is just being there. So here are some techniques I have seen work and some that don't work.

Reminiscing about the events and circumstances, if it's in agreement with the patient, is a powerful way of connecting: *Remember that family vacation when the tent collapsed? I will always remember how you dropped me off at college. Where were we when the car broke down in the middle of nowhere and we figured out how to change the tire? I loved that trip to Ireland with all the grandkids. Tell me about your childhood. Grandma always made the best banana bread.* You'll figure out what to say and how to start the conversation.

This is not the time to talk about the bankruptcy, the divorce, the brother you hated, or any type of negativity, but if the patient is heading in that direction, you may respectfully listen.

Some people have a greater connection to their pets than their families. With the input of the appropriate administration in a hospital or nursing home (most hospices welcome the family pet), that companion animal can often be brought to the bedside. This may require some creative maneuvering on the part of the family, but if we are reasonable about this and the pet is a traditional companion animal rather than some wild creature, this always can be a great source of comfort. If this isn't feasible, pictures of the pet placed on the wall or on the nightstand bring peace as well.

What happens to the beloved Labrador or Yorkie upon the death of the patient? This becomes an issue with many pet owners who need reassurance that someone will be finding the pet a new, loving home. Local animal shelters are particularly sensitive to placing pets whose owners have died. And many of these shelters are beneficiaries of memorials given on behalf of the pet owners.

Aromatherapy, oils, and massage can be powerful ways of connecting with the patient, if only to massage the hands and the feet with some appropriate oil. Peppermint seems to be healing. Don't feel obligated to do more than hold your loved one's hand if touching them makes you uncomfortable or seems inappropriate.

You should not sit on the bed without permission. Pull up a chair and just be there.

Usually at the bedside, one family member becomes the person in charge, directing the conversations, and that person needs to be acknowledged and listened to.

The dying process takes energy for the patient and can be fatiguing, and if this seems to be an issue, you should respectfully leave. Follow the lead of the main caregiver. Don't overstay your welcome.

Whether it's at home or in a hospice or hospital, the setting is less important than the atmosphere created by the family and close friends. Whether Grandma is dressed in her favorite flowered pajamas or Grandpa has photos of the "big one" caught on that Canadian fishing trip by his bedside, whether soothing music is playing or everyone takes a shift in just sitting by the bedside, almost always, it is these final death vigils that the families of patients remember.

What Dying People Say and Why They Say It

"My friend Steve was dying from liver cancer. He was weak and melting away before our eyes in the hospital bed. The doctor had arranged for him to go home that day with hospice care, and his wife, Martha, was packing the small bag when I arrived," my coauthor remembers.

"Martha filled me in out in the hallway. The prognosis was not good at all. Steve was quite aware of what came next: the confinement to bed because he was so weak, the morphine at home, a few days before he would be gone. I chose not to visit them at their home. This was their time. I would be intruding. So I leaned over the bed and wrapped him in a huge hug. The words stuck in my throat. I think I managed, 'Talk to you soon, Steve.'

"'I'm sorry,' he said.

"On the drive home, I kept wondering what he meant. Sorry for what?"

One of the end-of-life themes is being sorry. Saying "I'm sorry" can mean many things: sorry for never achieving personal greatness, sorry for moral transgressions, or sorry for putting the family through the illness. In Steve's case, he was probably sorry that he couldn't be there any longer, as a friend.

In my experiences at the bedside, I hear these phrases and more: "I screwed up." "If only…" "Always know that I care." "I apologize for the opportunities I missed to do the right thing."

If there is anything to learn from these poignant end-of-life confessions, it's that we all must find a way to live today so we have no regrets, no what-ifs, no if-onlys.

My colleague Dr. Ira Byock, a palliative expert, offers four phrases in his book, *The Four Things That Matter Most: A Book about Living,* that give us some lessons for what to say during that final embrace: "Please forgive me." "I forgive you." "Thank you." "I love you." He says these life-affirming phrases carry enormous power to mend and to nurture, at the end of life or in any relationship or life situation.

Greed (or Who Gets What)— Plain and Not So Simple

I do not pretend to have an MBA or to be an estate attorney, but we in the medical community do have some responsibility to at least make patients aware of the profound implications of wills, trusts, and financial planning. These dramas play out over the dying body more often than you can imagine. Then again, maybe you can.

I am astounded at how few patients have wills and how few of them understand the subtleties and nuances of estate planning, thereby forcing their families to sell assets to pay taxes and medical bills. Of course, this can cause tremendous ill will among survivors.

Money is *always* an underlying, if not overt, issue when families gather around a dying patriarch or matriarch. Without the proper wills and trusts and wise estate planning, the kids will squabble about the farm, the house, the cars, the retirement plans, the savings, the vacation home, the boat, the time-share, the jewelry, the coin collection, the heirlooms, and anything else of value.

I recall coming upon such a soap opera more than once. Adult children and spouses are sniping at each other while Grandpa shrinks away in his hospital bed, hooked up to all kinds of modern wonders, just prolonging the inevitable. Is anyone holding his hand and reminiscing? No, there's yelling, eyes rolling, hallway meetings that get somewhat loud.

At this point, I often approach the gathering at the bedside and say this: "Who has the most to gain when Grandpa dies?" Inevitably the group turns toward the eldest son, who will inherit the farm, or the daughter who has taken care of Grandpa for the past eight years. They all know what the will says. Groups of relatives line up like warring armies deciding who gets the spoils.

When money issues overshadow the dying process, this hardly provides enough sacred time to encourage the patient (who may not be able to participate at this point) to close the loop and connect on the difficult issues of sadness and sorrow and missed opportunities and fractured relationships. Moreover, it really does not allow the patient and the family to understand the crucial importance of estate planning and prudent legal advice during these difficult times.

When a patient is dying, it is hardly the ideal time to bring to the bedside the financial advisor, the accountant, and the estate attorney to sift through difficult issues of estate planning. I have seen this take place, especially when there is a large estate, business, or family farm that hasn't been resolved. I have also seen families bickering in the hallways, and even in the patient's hospital room, over Grandma's diamond ring or Grandpa's fishing tackle or Mom's antique pie plate or Dad's gold watch.

Some patients have not arranged for the orderly transfer of their financial assets. This can be disastrous, especially when there are second or third marriages as well as stepchildren and biological children, none of whom get along and each of whom has a hidden agenda—not to mention the agenda of in-laws, each of whom thinks they are entitled to the patient's estate.

A savvy social worker who helped me with the social aspects of end-of-life situations, Julie Assef, LSW, said, in her hospice experience, "Unfortunately, these fractures can linger for years after the patient's death, causing families to stop talking to each other and stop offering each other support in hard times. If people only knew the long-reaching impact of not leaving a clearly drawn will, more would make the effort early on."

Again, I'm not a lawyer or financial planner, but my own house is in order, and I have the lawyer bills to prove it. I review the arrangement often; I have just seen too many family feuds in the hospital hallways to want this for my own family.

20
Who Pulls the Plug?

WE DOCTORS REMEMBER SOME PEOPLE AND THEIR MEDICAL care as if we treated them yesterday. This is one of those for me. Susan was in her early fifties. She was a nonrecovering alcoholic, despite multiple evaluations and multiple inpatient treatments throughout the country.

She was admitted to the ICU with acute respiratory failure complicated by liver and kidney failure. She was sedated, had a respirator in place with a tracheal tube into the windpipe, was on dialysis for renal (kidney) failure, and was also on multiple antibiotics and other medications (called pressors) to maintain the blood pressure.

The respirator is the machine that breathes for the patient. If the patient has no spontaneous breathing, the respirator is programmed to push air into the lungs at periodic intervals. If the patient does have periodic episodes of breathing, the respirator pauses and allows the patient to breathe on their own.

The patient cannot talk with these tubes in place, and their hands are secured so they don't attempt to pull it out on their own. That's why these patients are lightly sedated.

Susan had been married but subsequently divorced and had a long-term relationship with a gentleman with whom she lived, although they were not married.

At the bedside were two adult brothers, and we were awaiting the arrival of her son, a law enforcement officer from Texas, who was driving to Minnesota. We had just a few days to make a life-or-death decision. The patient would have the breathing tube removed because, after about seven days, it causes a death of the cartilaginous tissue making up the windpipe, and then the patient is a candidate for a tracheostomy, which opens up all sorts of complications.

The scenario—and many others like it—goes something like this. Over the course of many consecutive days, we would have discussions at the bedside about the lack of benefit of continuing these aggressive interventions. It became clear that a decision needed to be made to take Susan off the ventilator, and none of the family members felt comfortable to do so. Since the patient was not married, there was no legal precedent as to who would make that decision. And Susan had not filled out an advance directive or named a healthcare proxy to act on her behalf.

We then arranged and scheduled a family meeting in a private conference room, where each of the medical team clearly identified themselves, and we understood who the major players were sitting around the table. The drama was complicated because we needed to await the arrival of the son. The patient's final wish before she was intubated was that she could be extubated (breathing tube removed) and express her regret to the family for her lifestyle.

Once the breathing tube is removed, most patients die within several hours, and we made that point very clear to the family. However, there are unusual circumstances where the patient would linger in a vegetative state for several weeks before finally dying. These are gut-wrenching decisions. This is a nightmare because most families believe that once the tube is removed, patients will quickly die. That is not always the case.

We also carefully explained that once the breathing tube was removed, we could not ascertain if Susan would have audible speech because of her weakened condition. Sadly, we could not even assure that she would be able to speak and express her regret to the family.

These discussions can take hours. We lay the groundwork. We discuss the medical situations in user-friendly, understandable terminology, not medical speak, and ask the family to ponder these options. We then revisit the following day.

The son arrived from Texas. In many cases, if it's not a son, it's an estranged daughter with a baby, or a long-lost brother. Families are complicated, and I'm not giving away any secrets here.

The patient was extubated, and she was able to verbalize her regret to the family. Despite the anguish and the tragedy of the situation, there were lots of hugs and acknowledgments for us on the medical side for our help, and what could have been a nightmare, in fact, had a happy, peaceful ending.

At some point in our lives most of us will spend time in an ICU (intensive care unit) or CCU (coronary care unit). Many individuals within thirty days of death will have this sort of intensive care that involves the technology of breathing machines, dialysis machines to cleanse the kidneys, as well as complex infusions of medications to treat infection, heart rhythm problems, and other bodily functions. In the ICU, by definition, patients are often treated by multiple levels of medical experts—most of whom know very little about the patient.

Once upon a time, when a patient was in one of these units, and if there was a difficult decision about the aggressiveness of care, the patient's primary care physician or internist or Marcus Welby, MD, could often be summoned to the bedside and act as an interpreter to help the patient and the family make the decision.

Today, however, we have the perfect storm of an aging American population, a transient population, who often become ill miles from home, a population who generally does not have a relationship with a primary physician, and a generation that typically does not write down their wishes. In general, 90 percent of us have not clearly spelled out what we want done to us or for us should we be in one of these complex situations.

A recent study by experts at the American Thoracic Society International Conference provided some chilling figures.

The frequency of having technology and support withdrawn reflected a sixfold variation, depending upon the intensive care unit. In some units, inappropriate life support was withdrawn from about 3 percent of patients; whereas, in other ICUs in other parts of the country, life support was taken away in up to 21 percent of patients.

In other words, whether or not life-sustaining treatments are withdrawn is a reflection on which intensive care unit the patient was in. If the patient does not have the capacity to express his or her wishes, it is the medical team, not the patient, who makes this decision in some states. In the absence of a designated healthcare proxy, your fate may be uncertain.

So an important lesson for each of us, when we are in the process of being admitted to one of the units, was to have spelled out clearly with our family and our significant others, but especially with the care team, the level of aggressiveness we want in our treatment. And if you are so ill or incapacitated (and many people often are) that you cannot speak for yourself at that time, let's hope your spouse or sister-in-law or daughter brings along a copy of your advance directive.

The culture of the ICU can be a major driver in aggressiveness of care. In some medical centers, there is a "win at all costs," cavalier, almost athletic military demeanor to sustain the patient with whatever means are necessary—even if this does not make sense and even if there is no reasonable probability of recovery. This is especially true when there is a young patient who may have experienced some traumatic event, such as a motorcycle accident, gunshot wound, or head trauma.

So, in these kinds of circumstances, that patient may be maintained in a persistent vegetative state with no probability of survival and no meaningful benefit.

On the other hand, there are some intensive care units that have a much less aggressive culture and are more willing to withdraw technical interventions, acknowledging that the situation is not reversible.

Please note that in each of these circumstances, the wishes of the patient and the family are certainly acknowledged, but a major factor in aggressiveness of care seems to be the prevailing culture or historical context of the intensive care unit.

The question, then, is this: How does a family know the ICU mentality? The short answer is, you don't. There are nuances of care that may not be fully known to the patient and family. If in a religious-oriented hospital—and historically every hospital came from a religious tradition—you may find the philosophical notion that life should be maintained at all costs, depending on the culture there. Now hospitals are more secular and motivated by healthcare profits. Heresy, you say? But something to consider, even if you have to have a talk with the hospital administrator about your concerns.

Consider Frank, a patient in his early seventies. A major outdoorsman. Frank had a leaky aortic valve in his heart, which was replaced by a senior surgeon. The surgery was flawless. The postoperative care was pristine; however, he did not awaken from anesthesia. Appropriate scans of the brain indicated massive brain injury from a series of strokes, which could not have been anticipated.

Frank's second wife was at the bedside. She was approximately half the age of the patient, and nearly the same age as the patient's daughters from marriage number one. As you can imagine, it was a volatile situation.

In conjunction with the surgical team, we made copies of the patient's operative report and carefully walked through the scenario with the family and explained that something unanticipated obviously happened during the operation.

A common scenario is to ask the family, "If Dad could awaken, if Frank could turn back the clock to his status of a month ago, what would he tell us to do?" Almost always, this alleviates the guilt of the family, and, under most circumstances, the patient is taken off life support systems and dies within several hours.

In another case, a prominent banker from a small community rolled his Harley on a rural county road and became a quadriplegic. Tom was a fit young man and could have been maintained in an artificial environment for years. We had a discussion in private and around the bedside asking his family what his wishes would have been. He was unable to speak and was not conscious, hooked up to life support systems.

There was a unanimous consensus that all support should be discontinued. He quietly passed away after several days, and the family was at peace.

And now we are back to the God issue. Doctors should not play God. We simply do not know how long a patient will live. Believe it or not, there are very few scientifically proven guidelines to predict a patient's short-term and long-term survival. Of course, there are clinical parameters that we all measure, such as blood levels of certain chemicals and certain findings on physical and neurological examination and the results of breathing studies and brain wave tests.

In real life when talking about death, these parameters are only rough guidelines and cannot provide a rigid number or percentage of survival for patients. Therefore, patients and families need to understand the importance of a dialogue, a conversation, a discussion about the reasonableness of aggressive care in a given patient's situation.

We each should designate a surrogate or a proxy or an individual who will express our wishes if we cannot express those wishes ourselves. This is the healthcare power of attorney or healthcare surrogate (someone to act on your behalf). It is different from an advance directive but works within it because the healthcare surrogate can assure that the patient's wishes are carried out.

Of course, it is important to have the written document, but it is also equally important to have a flowing discussion with that surrogate so that there is a clear understanding of your wishes and needs should you not be able to speak for yourself. It's not always binding if your mom told your dad while watching a medical show on TV one night, "I don't want to live like that. Just pull the plug. Promise me."

Let me explain how this process can go awry. Several years ago, a prominent celebrity, an athlete, was involved in a serious automobile accident with major head trauma. He had never started discussions about end-of-life decisions and had a complex domestic situation where his advisors included a business manager, a long-term domestic partner who did not have legal status, and a former partner who had been divorced from the celebrity.

When the primary care team discussed end-of-life issues with the family, it was not at all clear who the decision-maker was because of these complex legal and domestic entanglements. The decision about sustaining therapies became protracted, contentious, very public, and certainly increased the anguish of all relevant parties. We owe it to ourselves, and we also owe it to our families, to make our wishes crystal clear and to periodically review and update them to reflect changing life situations and relationships.

When the Plug Is Pulled

Once the decision has been made to discontinue mechanical intervention (to "unplug"), there is an orderly sequence that is followed. First, we eliminate medications that are not mission-critical for such things as pain management. Next, we wind down such therapies as IV fluids and kidney dialysis. And then, finally, the respirator is stopped. In some cases, the breathing tube is removed from the windpipe, and patients may pass away within several minutes. Some patients may linger for days after this process is completed. Other patients may lapse into a coma and die within several hours. We just don't know.

The medical team understands the anxiety of the patient during this time, if the patient is awake and aware. This is an hour-by-hour process. We clarify who will be around the bedside when the respirator is discontinued.

21

How Do We Resolve Ethical Dilemmas in Decision-Making for the Dying? The Role of the Advance Directive and Healthcare Proxy

VERN HAD FAR-ADVANCED LUNG CANCER. AT AGE SEVENTY-TWO, he found himself on a respirator and various opioids for pain and, as expected, with shortness of breath. He had articulated to his wife and to his social worker at the hospital that he wanted to be maintained with an artificial breathing machine and with kidney dialysis in this setting.

Now, seven days later, even though he was on a ventilator that prevented him from speaking, he was alert, and through eye contact and hand signals, he clearly indicated he wanted the dialysis discontinued and the breathing tube removed. In this setting, death would have followed within several hours if not within minutes.

Almost every patient from a palliative care perspective reflects profound ethical, legal, and moral issues. This is especially apparent if the patient does not have capacity. As explained previously, by capacity, we in medicine mean the ability, the executive cognitive functioning, to understand the pros, cons, risks, and benefits of a decision. This is very different from the legal term of competence. If patients are confused, if they are delusional, they cannot be expected to make clear decisions.

One of the cornerstones of medicine is autonomy, meaning to honor the wishes of the patient. However, our struggle was trying to understand if the patient indeed had capacity, since he was on a variety of medications. Did Vern really have capacity?

After thoughtful, in-depth, and gut-wrenching discussions with Vern and responsible family members, he was in agreement to continue with the current level of care. Several days later, he was safely extubated and did reasonably well until he succumbed to his advanced cancer.

The Advance Directive

The advance directive is actually a two-part legal document. The first part identifies a proxy or a surrogate or someone to speak on behalf of the patient if the patient is not able to speak for themselves because of illness. In general, this person is not the healthcare provider but is a spouse, partner, friend, confidant, or family member who is over eighteen and knows the patient well. This individual can make the "tough call" when it comes to speaking on behalf of the patient.

A spouse may be the proxy but not necessarily. Some people designate an adult child who is a nurse or a son or daughter or life partner or brother-in-law who may or may not be a healthcare professional.

The second equally important part of the document is to clearly outline what level of aggressiveness of care the patient desires if it is highly unlikely that the medical situation will improve. In this setting, the proxy would speak on behalf of the patient if the patient cannot clearly articulate their wishes.

In other words, if you were in a situation where there's no reasonable probability of benefit from a respirator or a feeding tube or dialysis, do you wish to be discontinued from technology that's prolonging your life? What might Vern's outcome have been if he had such a document?

There is a lot of confusion about the mechanics of this document. Every healthcare institution has this document on hand, and usually the wording is very easy to understand and not at all complicated.

You do not need the input or guidance of an attorney to execute this form. In general, a patient would fill out the form, usually in the setting of two witnesses, one of whom may be the healthcare provider, such as the physician or nurse. These two witnesses document that the person filling out the form is indeed the patient.

The other option is to have the form notarized, and this is easily done, since notaries are available in every healthcare institution. Ideally, the document is filled out well in advance of any dire medical situation.

We obviously have no idea what today or tomorrow may hold for us, but, for the peace of mind of our family, it is crucial that we have a properly executed advance directive and designated proxy to speak for us.

However, life is not simple, and problems arise. Each state has specific guidelines about these documents, and it is important if you have a residence in multiple states that you make some inquiry as to the local policies and procedures in order to make certain that the advance directive is up-to-date and in force, whether you're wintering in Florida or boating in Minneapolis in summer.

Now on a more personal note, my wife and I typically review our advance directives every year or so. We indicate that if the weight of medical judgment clearly indicates that it is not reasonable to anticipate an improvement from a current situation, we would not wish to be maintained on machines, but we would want a "full court press" in terms of quality of life and sense of well-being.

These documents in general should be scanned into our medical record and kept with us, especially when we travel, so there is a clear understanding of what our wishes are when faced with these life-transforming events. Some people keep these scanned as images on their smartphones or in the cloud for easy access.

One of our patients, Harold, had an artificial heart. So he was seriously compromised to begin with. He was admitted to the hospital with an overwhelming bloodstream infection. He required kidney dialysis. He required medications to maintain his blood pressure and pulse, and it was clear after weeks in this situation that it was improbable that he would ever recover. He was not awake or aware or able to participate in his care.

The family was profoundly supportive at the bedside vigil day after day and insisted that this aggressive care be continued. Despite multiple family conferences and input from other professionals, including clergy, the family would "not give up," and the patient was sustained in this situation for months. Without knowing what Harold would have wanted, his family made the decisions, and, frankly, this is not what I would have chosen for myself.

Harold's case is an extreme example of the kinds of challenges that the palliative care team faces. Without input and guidance, patients and their families are overwhelmed by the complexity of care. In many institutions, we on the medical care team are viewed as providing some element of continuity while trying to provide clarity for patients and families during a time of chaos.

In almost every palliative care consultation, we acknowledge the hierarchy of decision-making for patients who do not have the capacity to express their own wishes because of, for example, a head injury, stroke, or some other medical condition, like Harold's.

If a healthcare proxy was not named by the patient, a close family member or friend could step up and speak on behalf of the patient. Alternatively, there may be an individual not related to the patient, who, for a variety of reasons, feels comfortable with and is acknowledged by the family as having the legitimacy to speak on behalf of the patient.

Under some circumstances, there is a court-ordered surrogate, but this is a clumsy and time-consuming process. Usually, with reasonableness, more appropriate avenues can be taken.

A difficult situation arises for the patient who never had capacity by virtue of a birth injury or some other situation, and there are strong protectors in place to protect the rights of these individuals. These protectors typically come from the ranks of mental health and social work. In some cases, a social worker may be able to contact an acquaintance of a homeless patient, for example, who has an idea of the patient's wishes. The friend would be asked if the patient ever talked about this type of situation. These are always difficult to resolve.

Wouldn't life (and death) be a lot less guilt ridden if the patient had provided some guidance in the form of a well-thought-out, written document and considered the issues long before a medical crisis put everyone inside the tornado?

In the resources section of this book, I have provided links to websites where you can download and execute these vital documents. I encourage you to do so. Now is the right time.

A Partnership with Patient Rights and Caregiver Responsibilities

Almost every encounter at the end of life, or anywhere along the journey of a patient with serious illness, raises ethical, moral, and almost theological concepts. Patients and families need to have some understanding of these issues, or there can be a tremendous misunderstanding.

Patients and families can expect these core values from the palliative care team:

- Relief of suffering rather than prolongation of life

- A supportive, caring environment for the patient rather than simply treating a disease or a condition, such as congestive heart failure or emphysema

- Attention and respect for the values and the cultural imperatives of the patient and the family rather than imposing the values of the care team

- Recognizing, embracing, and working with the existential and spiritual issues of the patient and family rather than imposing those of the care team

- Enlisting a concept of a therapeutic partnership and collaborative relationship rather than a dictatorial, one-sided relationship where the physician and other caregivers dictate to the patient

Then there is the question about the course of treatment. We on the medical team understand that patients have rights and responsibilities, but they do not have the right to demand treatment that in the view of the professional would not be beneficial. For example, it is customary that surgeons may not agree to operate on a patient, and it is certainly common practice that some oncologists would not endorse or support a certain line of treatment even if so insisted upon by the patient. Let me explain.

Sylvia was a seventy-seven-year-old, frail, elderly widow who had far-advanced breast cancer. She had progressed through three types of standard chemotherapy and was in a highly weakened condition. She was bedfast for more than half of her waking hours and had lost approximately 10 percent of her body weight within the previous six months.

Both Sylvia and her adult daughter insisted vehemently on a fourth line of chemotherapy. The medical team explained the absence of convincing evidence for benefit and declined the patient's request, but we offered to help her get another medical opinion. So, under highly specific circumstances, the care team may appropriately refuse the patient's request for treatment.

Now, this leads us into discussion of "medical futility." Futility used in the medical environment is difficult to define. However, much like art and athleticism, we know it when we see it.

As a generally accepted concept, if a certain treatment showed no benefit in the last 100 cases, it seems highly improbable that patient 101 would have results that were positive from the intervention. During these painful encounters with patients and families, there also needs to be a frank discussion of the benefits and burdens of the proposed treatment.

The medical team is often pulled into these discussions because the patient's grandson read about a promising treatment on the internet or heard about some far-away medical center conducting a clinical trial in phase 1 of study for a similar condition. Or a well-meaning neighbor or coworker brings up treatments in no way related to the disease condition at hand. And then we are all running down a rabbit hole of futility.

Franklin, at age fifty-five, was morbidly obese, with high blood pressure and diabetes. He was actively dying from congestive heart failure. He could barely speak a sentence. He needed help to get out of bed and was unable to walk without assistance.

In this desperate situation, his family asked about a heart transplant. Would he be a good candidate? Would a transplant help? We appropriately counseled about the obvious risks of a heart transplant in someone so compromised, and when this was done in a thoughtful, compassionate manner, the patient and family withdrew that request.

The Needs of the Patient Come First

The mantra of Mayo Clinic is this: "The only need to be considered is the need of the patient."

In other words, the needs of the patient come first. This was articulated by Dr. Charles Mayo at a commencement address at Rush Medical School in the early 1900s. This concept is embedded into the soul of every employee at Mayo Clinic, from the entry-level worker to the leadership of the organization.

Now when we come to the critically ill patient who can verbalize their wishes, the decision-making process becomes straightforward. The patient's wishes must be honored and acknowledged, even if the wishes of that patient are in conflict with that of the family. I have discussed these types of conflicts in the section on family meetings. But if the patient cannot verbalize their wishes, the issue becomes extremely complicated.

If the patient cannot verbalize their wishes, an important and helpful technique would be the family conference asking this question I have mentioned many times, "If Dad (or Mom) could awaken from this state and be off of the respirator, and if he (or she) had fifteen minutes of being lucid and engaged, what do you think, from your knowledge of the patient, that he (or she) would share with us?"

This helps the medical team and the family focus on the patient's wishes. What we often hear is something like this: "Dad has been an avid hunter or fisherman" or "Mom loved to garden and care for her grandkids." And then we hear that if these options were not realistic for the patient, they would not want to be sustained artificially with tubes and devices and machines.

So, by thoughtfully discussing what the patient would wish, based upon previous lifestyle choices, the decision becomes fairly straightforward. It is often not without anguish and confrontation, but this technique frequently provides clarity to help the family make a decision consistent with the patient's past wishes—in the absence of an advance directive.

Responsibilities and Fears of the Healthcare Surrogate

In an ideal situation, which hardly never occurs, the patient has a clearly written advance directive in which the patient indicates the proxy or surrogate decision-maker, should the patient not be able to speak for themselves, and also stipulates the aggressiveness of care that that patient requires.

However, situations are dramatically complicated. The surrogate, under some circumstances, can act without following the advance directive. Let me explain. Advance directives often state something to the effect that if the patient were in a situation where the probability of cure was low, the patient would not wish to be intubated or undergo kidney dialysis. This is clear, but let me present an all-too-common scenario.

The patient has an advance directive in place and has been healthy but then has, let's say, an automobile accident or a traumatic event where aggressive intubation and kidney dialysis may offer that patient the possibility of recovering from this situation. Well, if the surrogate followed the precise wording of the patient's advance directive, the surrogate would not allow intubation or renal dialysis. However, with careful counseling to reverse the patient's wishes, the surrogate in this situation is acting in the patient's best interest because intubation and renal dialysis might give that patient the probability of recovery from this event.

In other words, the proxy can apply "substituted judgment" to make a decision on behalf of the patient, acting in the patient's best interests.

Then we have the surrogate who will not be able to follow the directive. Consider the husband and wife who have been married for fifty-plus years. Each is the healthcare proxy for the other. He has a stroke. He's intubated and languishing in the ICU. The doctors say his brain bleed has taken over half his brain. There is no relevant brain activity. Can she carry out his wishes for no heroic measures, and disconnect him?

Judy, a nurse, whose husband this is describing, told me, "As a retired nurse, I knew he was facing a cascading number of medical problems, and he already had failing kidneys and was diabetic. The renal doctor offered to start dialysis. My brain was divided—the nurse brain on one side and the wife brain on the other. I knew medically that his quality of life, which he valued, would be almost nonexistent, and from that point of view my decision was easy. As his wife, though, my heart wanted to desperately hang on to him and not say goodbye. One of my friends reminded me later that I gave him a great gift."

These are the real-life scenarios you never consider when you're signing such documents as advance directives. The what-ifs intervene. In these cases, the wife might consult with adult children about "what Dad might want," and the family meeting then becomes a crucial decision-making process as the family works through the anguishing dilemma.

Another option would be to review the advance directive and proxy every few years with an eye toward such situations. Perhaps switch the proxy to an adult child a parent feels might make less emotional but equally weighty decisions. Every family is different.

Some people designate two people as their healthcare proxies. I'm not sure this is the greatest idea because if they disagree, the document is not going to be helpful. The key is to decide to use the word *and*, meaning they must act together; or, *or*, meaning they may act independently.

The bottom line for me is to have these open discussions with your family at the dinner table. That's where the world's problems are resolved anyway. Back up the consensus with a current advance directive and healthcare proxy, and make sure the surrogate knows their designation as such and has a copy of the document.

22

Can You Help Me Understand the Advance Directive?

LET'S SAY YOU ARE SITTING IN THE LAWYER'S OFFICE WITH A printed document in front of you. You're about to decide what you want in an end-of-life situation, after which two witnesses and a notary are going to validate your document.

Is that the best setting to make those decisions? I think not.

My suggestion is to get a copy of the blank advance directive document for your state. (The resources section of this book lists websites where you can download an advance directive for your state.) Read the document, make notes, discuss your wishes with your spouse or partner or friend, and certainly with the person who is going to be designated as your healthcare power of attorney or surrogate or proxy.

Give yourself time to reflect on what you want. As I often say, if you're arrested for drunk driving, that's not the time to start looking online for a lawyer.

After you've reviewed the document, reflected on your wishes, and had the necessary conversations with the pertinent people, fill out your document and have the appropriate witnesses and notary attest to your signature. Make copies for your surrogate and your medical file at your doctor's office, and keep a copy with you. Some elderly people are encouraged to keep this document in an envelope on the back of their front door (presumably for

911 responders, but they will not read it; they will do all they can to resuscitate you).

From South Dakota and Minnesota to Texas and from California to New York, the advance directives take many forms and offer a variety of questions, but some questions are fairly universal.

Let me offer general questions here and discuss what patients often answer, how families and specifically the healthcare power of attorney or surrogate should interpret those responses, and what we on the medical team understand about those answers.

Some states will ask you to respond to questions like this:

- If I had a reasonable chance of recovery, and were temporarily unable to decide or speak for myself, I would want:

- If I were dying and unable to decide or speak for myself, I would want:

- If I were permanently unconscious and unable to decide or speak for myself, I would want:

- If I were completely dependent on others for my care and unable to decide or speak for myself, I would want:

- In all circumstances, my doctors will try to keep me comfortable and reduce my pain. This is how I feel about pain relief if it would affect my alertness or if it could shorten my life:

Other states ask for a straightforward yes or no to questions like this:

□ **Choose NOT to Prolong Life.** I do not want my life to be prolonged if (1) I have an incurable and irreversible condition that will result in my death within a relatively short time, (2)

I become unconscious and, to a reasonable degree of medical certainty, I will not regain consciousness, or (3) the likely risks and burdens of treatment would outweigh the expected benefits.

OR

◻ **Choose to Prolong Life.** I want my life to be prolonged as long as possible within the limits of generally accepted health-care standards.

As seen earlier, you may be asked about relief from pain, even if it hastens your death.

Some forms may give you many choices and an option to write out your own wishes. You decide how much detail to put in the document. You might say this:

- If my death is imminent, I choose not to prolong my life. If life-sustaining treatment has been started, stop it, but keep me comfortable and control my pain.

  OR

- Even if my death is imminent, I choose to prolong my life.

  OR

- I choose neither of the above options, and here are my instructions should I become terminally ill and my death is imminent: [add your specifics here].

You may be asked about artificial nutrition and hydration through a feeding tube inserted into the stomach or through a needle in a vein:

- If my death is imminent, I do not want artificial nutrition and hydration. If it has been started, stop it.

OR

- Even if my death is imminent, I want artificial nutrition and hydration.

If, in the judgment of my physician, I am suffering with a *terminal condition* from which I am expected to die within six months, even with available life-sustaining treatment provided in accordance with prevailing standards of medical care:

- I request that all treatments other than those needed to keep me comfortable be discontinued or withheld, and my physician will allow me to die as gently as possible.

OR

- I request that I be kept alive in this terminal condition, using available life-sustaining treatment.

If, in the judgment of my physician, I am suffering with an *irreversible condition* so that I cannot care for myself or make decisions for myself and am expected to die without life-sustaining treatment provided in accordance with prevailing standards of care:

- I request that all treatments other than those needed to keep me comfortable be discontinued or withheld, and my physician will allow me to die as gently as possible.

OR

- I request that I be kept alive in this irreversible condition, using available life-sustaining treatment.

Option 1 (choosing not to prolong life) is an ideal situation, which quite honestly almost never occurs. The terminology in these documents is ambiguous, and most families don't really know what the patient meant. However, if option 1 contains the term "no reasonable probability of improvement," then the patient's wishes are clear, and everyone is at peace.

A true case. Several years ago, I cared for a prominent baseball personality who had a cardiac arrest at spring training. Because of Minnesota connections, he was evacuated to Minnesota on my service. Around the bedside was his grieving wife and three adult children who were household names in the baseball world. When queried as to the patient's wishes, no one had a clue. The family was devastated.

The next day, they looked completely different. The wife had gone through a safe-deposit box and came across a handwritten note by the patient stating that if he was not going to get better, he would not want any of these interventions. Care was de-escalated, and everyone felt good about that decision.

At some point, the artificial interventions are deemed to be of no benefit and are no longer deemed to be life-sustaining, because of complications. As mentioned, the word *futility* is now never used because it is too hard to define. If the family wishes measures to be continued indefinitely, an ethics consultation or a court order might be reached, but this is a rare circumstance.

Consider the people you leave behind and their anguish in making these bedside decisions. Then execute an advance directive.

23

Who Are the Players around the Bed?

I'VE MENTIONED DR. FRANK, OUR BELOVED FAMILY PHYSICIAN in our community just outside New York City in the 1950s and 1960s. He made house calls with his tattered leather bag, out of which he pulled a few instruments, such as a stethoscope and a reflex hammer.

As soon as he walked into the room, there was a sense of peace and comfort: we would say, "Dr. Frank is here," and we believed that everything would be fine. He was always paid in cash. There was no paper trail. There was no insurance.

The Family Doc

Once upon a time, the relationship between the patient and the physician was a one-on-one encounter. The patient came with a health concern; the physician recommended treatments for the patient; the treatments were carried out, and that was the end of the story. Today, however, the situation has dramatically changed.

Incredibly complex and unbelievably expensive interventions, such as the CT scan, have evolved. The MRI and the PET scans have since followed. These interventions require the financial input of insurance companies, and this changed everything. Insurance companies are now among the players around the bed and inside the exam room.

When I approach the bedside of a patient who is hospitalized—and who clearly has a serious medical problem simply by virtue of being in the hospital—the patient and the family need to understand that around the bedside are a number of other stakeholders who clearly impact the well-being of the patient.

The Insurance Company

Like it or not (mostly not), the insurance company, the hospital administrator, the chair of the division or the department in which the physician works, and a whole array of state, regional, and federal regulators, each of whom has a stake in the management of that patient, all are at the bedside—not literally, of course, but the presence of each of them is felt. So let me give you a practical example.

Several years ago, I was caring for a wonderful gentleman who had a serious cancer that continued to worsen through a number of types of standard and investigative chemotherapies. Through an extensive search of the literature, we then became aware of a program that would offer potential promise for this patient. This particular injection was generally accepted by practitioners as being safe and reasonable, but it had not received official FDA endorsement. That endorsement is usually the gold standard for insurance companies to reimburse the patient for the treatment.

Following the guidelines that the needs of the patient come first, we had multiple discussions with the insurance company, with appropriate documentation that this particular treatment was viewed as standard even though it did not have the official seal of the FDA. After months of hassles, the insurance company finally agreed to reimburse the patient for the treatment.

This is what I mean by many stakeholders around the bedside. Patients and families need to understand that if a treatment or a procedure is not supported by the insurance company, there is an appeals process. But let me be very clear: this can be an exhausting, laborious, and time-consuming process, as well as a bureaucratic nightmare.

So how can we finesse the system? Here is a "cookbook" that patients and families can use:

- Obviously, there needs to be written documentation, typically from the healthcare provider to the insurance company, explaining why the treatment or procedure is necessary. This sort of letter must be accompanied by documentation, either from the literature or from clinical experience, as to why this treatment should be supported.

- Almost predictably, the letter will be rejected, or it will be lost. So the patient, the family, and the physician need to have the name, the title, and the phone number for the patient advocate in the insurance company who acts as a case manager. These individuals themselves do not actually make any decisions, but they are important allies to have. Contact them.

- If there is no appropriate resolution of the dilemma, there needs to be a direct communication with the medical director of the insurance company (these are doctors who oversee these types of requests). Patients obviously do not have the necessary knowledge or experience to effectively address concerns with the medical director; this is where the patient's physician or care team comes into play.

- From my own experience, most medical directors are reasonable, and most do want to do the right thing on behalf of the patient. I have found that to enlist their support in a collegial and professional manner, as opposed to an adversarial one, will usually open doors and possibilities.

- There is little merit in becoming confrontational, even though it's our instinct to do so, but there is great merit in including that medical director in a treatment plan.

This process can be complex and will often siphon off lots of energy, so the patient needs that friend, that advocate, that family member who understands the importance of tenacity and resilience in dealing with some of these issues.

One of the real problems is that there are too many cooks in the insurance kitchen, and it is sometimes difficult to identify that key person in the insurance company who is qualified and empowered to make a decision. Often these somewhat experimental treatments are so new that we don't know the outcomes. I describe the efforts almost as a "Hail Mary" football pass. Just considering them is a subject for that all-important family meeting described in an earlier chapter.

Another issue that patients and families need to understand is the out-of-network situation. Most patients have insurance coverage that will absorb most of the costs of treatment, which is given by a selected group of providers typically in their community. If, for some reason, the patient uses an out-of-network provider or facility, the patient is responsible for a greater proportion of the bill. Let me give you an example.

A beloved family member lives in another state and has a complex medical problem. The specific specialist most qualified to deal with the patient's problem was not an in-network provider. Using an out-of-network provider would result in the patient having to pay the full cost. There can be tremendous misunderstandings if these issues are not clarified up front, so the patient needs to have that name and phone number of the insurance representative who can clarify who pays for what.

Many patients would share with me, "Doc, no problem; we have an 80/20 policy." This means that the company picks up 80 percent of the bill, and the patient is responsible for the remaining 20 percent. But this is not the entire story. It is not at all uncommon for a bill to be hundreds of thousands of dollars. Twenty percent of a $200,000 medical bill is still $40,000, and that is a significant outlay, even for a patient with substantial resources.

When patients are ill, sick, and frightened, these kinds of issues are hardly on their radar screen. Nevertheless, they cannot be ignored, even though paying bills is the last task any desperately ill patient cares about.

When the patient dies, the mountain of final and past-due bills coming to the estate's executor—presumably a family member—can be overwhelming. There may be bills from the hospital, from the clinic, as well as from independent contractors who provide services but are not part of the formal medical staff, specialists, the physical therapist, the anesthesiologist, certain physician extenders, in-network providers, out-of-network providers, medical equipment companies for oxygen and tube feedings, hospice, ambulance services, and others.

As in most circumstances of life, there really is no substitute for that personal discussion with a live human (face-to-face or by phone) on complex billing and insurance issues. Visit the hospital's billing department or the nursing home's financial officer while you're there. Navigating impersonal voice-mail hell to reach someone empowered to help within insurance companies or in providers' billing offices is guaranteed to try anyone's patience.

The best advice from others who have been there is to keep careful notes about who said what, the date, and their contact information. Email, although impersonal, is your tracking of who said what. Don't give up. Some providers can write off certain medical costs to charity care. Sometimes it's prudent to turn over those tasks to estate lawyers or accountants.

An Outside Caregiver

Sometimes outside caregivers become part of the care team at the bedside. Although my experience with patients is in a hospital setting, where the visitors are family and close friends, when a gravely ill person goes home with hospice—or just goes home—the family may hire outside caregivers to be at the bedside.

Why? For a number of reasons: family members need a break; there may be no nearby family members to provide care; the type of care requires some nursing skills; round-the-clock care is needed; or it's simply the preference of the patient or the family. I'm sure there are more reasons, and that's why many of these in-home companion companies are doing so well.

I can tell you what I have heard. Many home-care companies supply a series of temporary workers with little formal training in dealing with end-of-life issues. In general, these bedside companions are high-priced babysitters. Most are poorly prepared to handle any urgent issues. In addition, you pay a high hourly fee, while the hapless caregiver is paid something closer to minimum wage.

Julie told us about her mother's experience, where an eight-year decline with dementia proved to be a nightmare for the family: "Our biggest challenge was daily care at home. After hip surgery, the insurance company was pressuring me to take her home." And thus began the parade of caregivers "from highly recommended agencies."

She described how "they stole from us, ignored my mother to do schoolwork (many were nursing or college students), talked on their cell phones. They broke things. They wasted food and resources. It was insane, stressful, and expensive."

In my own family, my wife's brother was profoundly demented, so we could not leave him alone at home where his wife was handling the bulk of the caregiving. To give her a break for personal and business needs, the family asked around in their midsized community to find a caregiver to stay on occasion.

Sometimes the only recourse is word of mouth, because I know there are compassionate and trained companions available. Maybe this is one of the best uses for a post on Facebook or other social media platforms. Be sure to get and talk to references, find out the going hourly rate, and meet the person face-to-face. Consider a "nanny cam" (hidden video camera) if you really want to be vigilant, but this raises all kinds of privacy and confidentiality issues, so beware.

The Unwanted Visitor (Virtually and Otherwise)

In most circumstances, around the bed is the patient's spouse, partner, or longtime friend; adult children; and grandchildren, depending upon their ages. Siblings and their spouses, along with in-laws, are also familiar visitors. Clergy, if invited, are familiar visitors.

But what about Aunt Beulah, who shows up unexpectedly with an entourage of cousins? A nosy neighbor, church acquaintances, the mah jongg girls, the bridge club—you get the idea. Causing unneeded angst could be the estranged ex-wife, the bookie, the angry business partner, a disinherited daughter, a disenfranchised alcoholic brother-in-law, and any number of people who would not be welcome at this sacred time. The bedside at the end of life is not the place for added drama, as I have continually described throughout this book.

Someone in the close family needs to be in charge to disinvite unwanted visitors and almost literally bar the door. Under some circumstances, the family lawyer could get involved in keeping people away. A sign could be placed on the door indicating the patient inside is under hospice care.

How do these unwanted visitors find out about the situation? It's obvious the role social media are playing. Everything becomes public. The family may want to appoint just one person to handle family messaging on a private basis. But without some filters, every blood test or bowel movement becomes public knowledge with one simple Facebook or Instagram post.

Those of us on the medical team do not want our every consultation and quotation shared. These messages can be taken out of context like a bad game of whispered telephone. We would not like our bedside consultations or family meetings videotaped or streamed, because this raises questions of patient confidentiality.

Surely, there are enough players around the bedside without adding to the turmoil.

24
What about
Physician-Assisted Suicide?

BRINKLEY WAS ILL. OLD AND ILL. HE HAD LIVED A LONG, productive life as a therapist. His patients loved him. He was at their bedside, and unspoken words sent his healing message to more patients than I can count. But, as a result of cancer, his organs were failing. His kidneys were shutting down. It was just a matter of days.

My wife, Peggy, and I were there when the doctor injected Brinkley with the medicine that would stop his heart. As Brinkley slipped away, as his heart stopped, our hearts broke. Brinkley was our beloved dog. We had rescued him from a local animal shelter. He had only three legs after one was amputated from a severe injury as a puppy. And he had rescued us with years of unconditional love. He became an uncertified therapy dog at a local retirement facility, and he visited patients and their families countless times.

We've all faced this common gut-wrenching dilemma. That cherished pet, perhaps a dog or a cat who is not doing well, is obviously suffering from some condition—whether it be medical or traumatic—and there is no reasonable probability of recovery. Our pet is then taken to the veterinarian, and after anguishing decisions, the animal, the faithful family friend, is quietly put to sleep.

Now the logical extension of this painful situation brings us to the bedside. We in the palliative care world repeatedly hear something like this: "Well, if we can put our dog or cat out of its misery, why can't we extend the same thought process to patients?" "My father-in-law is suffering. I wouldn't let my dog suffer like that."

Let's start this conversation because this is clearly on the radar screen of almost every family member dealing with a relative with a serious end-of-life situation.

The states of Oregon and Washington, and others, through general elections have endorsed and supported the notion of physician-assisted suicide or physician-assisted death. More recently, Vermont has become the first state to legalize this procedure through the state legislature and legislative process. So what does this really mean, and what do we need to know about physician-assisted death?

For starters, there are some important distinctions. First, let's focus on euthanasia. This is the deliberate, intentional, and willful ending of a patient's life by a healthcare provider, and this typically consists of a lethal injection. This is not legal in any state in the US.

Now let's turn to the issue of physician-assisted suicide, more commonly described in ethical circles as physician-assisted death. This concept consists of the physician or healthcare provider sharing with the patient the education, the needs, and the methods to take their own life.

How does that work? Under some circumstances, the physician will prescribe a barbiturate such as Seconal, which the patient or family member will pick up at a drugstore. There are then clear instructions of how that medication is mixed with a slurry drink that the patient swallows. The dose is deliberately designed to end the patient's life. This technique has been legalized in the states that I mentioned.

Let's look at the historical context of this situation. The Netherlands has led the way in these techniques. If a patient had a desperate situation and requested physician-assisted suicide, and if two physicians were in agreement, then, legally, that patient could enlist the help of those providers to end their own life.

You will recall the controversy surrounding Dr. Jack Kevorkian, a pathologist who was known for helping patients (at least 130) die. He was convicted of murder in 1999 and served time in prison. His public stance on a patient's right to die using physician-assisted suicide kick-started reform in this area.

But now this leads us into the concept of a slippery slope. Initially, there were clear guidelines. The patient had to be of sound mind and judgment; the patient needed to be completely with capacity to understand the implications of their decision. However, as you can easily imagine, there has been a softening of these guidelines, and there now are concerns that some patients will participate in physician-assisted suicide and not really understand the implications of their actions.

In the Netherlands, the issue of physician-assisted suicide has been prime-time news. We have read reports of individuals who do not have a terminal illness being euthanized—and, under some circumstances, without their consent. When guidelines are loosened, decisions are made for convenience.

We need to understand that these are not simply theoretical concerns but practical daily issues that we cannot ignore. With the aging of the American population, with the breakup and subtle disintegration of family and community and religious ties, and with the isolation of many members of our community, it is not difficult to envision circumstances where patients might be offered these options for economic considerations. Consider the greedy nephew or other scam artist who gets a gravely ill elderly woman (maybe someone with no immediate family) to sign over all assets "because I love you."

So we need to be painfully aware that it is not reasonable to extrapolate from the veterinary environment, where the faithful family friend is put to sleep, to the bedside that involves a human patient.

Extensive literature assessing the backgrounds of patients who request physician-assisted suicide is very clear. One of the most common reasons for patients to request this intervention is the perception of lack of control over their lives and the fear of being a burden to their families. Interestingly, the issue of pain is relatively low on the list. So, if patients feel engaged with their healthcare provider, feel validated and acknowledged, and share in the management of their condition, these requests will become infrequent and ultimately vanish.

Within the past decade the concept of "death panel" was mentioned in some political circles, and I can vividly recall a small number of elderly patients referring to this issue and wondering if their age would be a factor in determining the appropriateness of their care (it doesn't). Likewise, some individuals with developmental and physical disabilities were fearful that, because of economic pressures and now the legalization of physician-assisted death, they might be at risk (they are not).

Now, a logical extension of these discussions clearly focuses on the issue of intentionality and the concept of double effect. If morphine is provided to the patient to relieve such symptoms as shortness of breath, air hunger, or pain, and if a well-recognized and an acknowledged side effect of the medication might be a slowing of breathing and a slowing of the heart but the intent is to decrease pain and shortness of breath, that is a morally acceptable intervention without any legal consequences.

It is absolutely crucial that providers clearly articulate to the patient and the family the intent, the potential side effects, and the likely ultimate outcome of administering morphine and similar medications. In other words, the intent of the medications, the intent of the intervention, is to enhance quality of life; however, an accepted and recognized side effect is that the patient may have labored breathing and a slow heart rate resulting in their death. Nevertheless—and this is the key point to emphasize—the patient's death was not the intent of the treatment.

With the ever-deepening complexity and ever-increasing cost of medical treatments, and with the aging of the American population, we all need to participate in these conversations so that we can be informed and knowledgeable in dealing with crucial end-of-life discussions—for our loved ones and eventually for ourselves.

25

How Do We Help in Grieving for Life and Loss?

VICKI WAS DIAGNOSED WITH COLON CANCER, AND ONCE THE standard course of chemotherapy failed to provide the cure we all expected, she was accepted into a clinical trial, and then another, all to no avail. The cancer cells kept mutating and eluding the powerful chemicals designed to kill them. But this is not a story about mutant cancer cells. This is the story about the type of cancer patient we all admire for her incredible courage as bad news just kept coming her way.

She informed her growing number of Facebook followers that she was arming up with red lipstick for each new chemo session. The red lipstick emoji became her battle cry and that of her loyal tribe. When good news came in the form of encouraging lab results, she'd get the chemo nurses (even the guys) to wear red lipstick and post pictures in celebration. Instead of trying to find ways to boost her spirits, her friends said that Vicki was boosting theirs with her red lipstick campaign.

If you've worked in the medical field as long as I have and with the thousands of patients and their families, with pain and suffering every day—because as a cancer doctor my patients don't always have miraculous outcomes—you cannot discount the interaction of the mind, the body, the spirit, and the soul. Attitude and disposition and the way we view the world have a tremendous impact on how we deal with serious illness.

The concept of *spirituality* means different things to different people. A working definition that we commonly use in the palliative care arena, borrowed from a wise chaplain working with our team, is that spirituality is an inner search for meaning and purpose, especially in the face of chaos and uncertainty.

On the other hand, the concept of *religion* usually implies the rules and the regulations and the ceremonies around the belief system. For example, the Catholic tradition would involve Mass and going to confession and receiving the holy Eucharist as part of church rules and rituals. Spirituality, on the other hand, is a more personal inner belief system.

In my clinical experience, almost every patient at the moment of crisis reaches out for a reassuring mosque, a sweat lodge, a synagogue, a church, a place of worship—this is a form of reaching out to some transcendental power or factor, whether named or unnamed, to provide peace and consolation during these difficult times.

Vicki, by example, reached out to her friends and family and wrapped herself in a profound spirituality of friendship and community—a "we're all in this together" bond signified by red lipstick. Her celebration-of-life party was punctuated with red lipstick, tears, and hugs. And the deep spirituality of her life brought people together in their grief.

We cannot forget the classic book by Holocaust survivor Viktor Frankl entitled *Man's Search for Meaning*. Dr. Frankl was an Austrian-born psychiatrist imprisoned at Auschwitz, in the midst of the horror. He made a mental note of why some prisoners survived and others did not. The individuals with a sense of meaning and purpose and connectedness, typically driven by relationships, somehow were among those few people who survived the camps. The individuals who survived had that inner sense of belief and recognized the importance of attitude and disposition in dealing with adversity.

A real challenge that we in palliative medicine face in the hospital is when patients and families are at different places in their psychological and spiritual journeys. Here's an example.

Joseph was a fifty-six-year-old farmer with far-advanced cancer of the pancreas, which had spread to his liver and bones. He was deeply jaundiced. His liver was deteriorating, and traditional chemotherapy and radiation had not stemmed the tide of this dreadful illness. He told the medical team that he was ready to let go. He had fought the good fight. He had mended fences. He had closed chapters. He was prepared to move on to the next phase and quietly pass away.

As often happens, many family members, including his spouse, were on a much different train on a much different track. They tenaciously held on to the hope that some other institution and some other surgeon and some other physician would have a magical medicine, a potion, an elixir to make this cancer go away.

This dichotomy between where the patient is and where the family is can be a source of great stress for everyone. One of the roles of the palliative team is to compassionately educate the patient and family as to the reality of the situation, never completely shutting the door on hope but also bringing the family to the point where they recognize that a cure is not possible and the focus should be placed on quality of life and sense of well-being.

The Myth of Not Battling Hard Enough

During the mid-1980s, Bernie Siegel's book *Love, Medicine, and Miracles: Lessons Learned about Self-Healing from a Surgeon's Experience with Exceptional Patients* appeared in hospital rooms throughout the United States. This was an important work because it discussed patient involvement in dealing with cancer. He championed a heightened sense of responsibility. He encouraged patients to be active participants in treatment decisions. Patients were appropriately invited to challenge the medical institution itself and were advised not to be passive participants swept away by the armada of medical technology.

Eventually, this positive message became distorted. Some authors suggested that the "fighters"—patients who tenaciously engaged their doctors in alternative practices—and the "opti-mists" would somehow be granted a reprieve from their illness.

This misguided philosophy placed a dreadful burden on the shoulders of each patient. I saw this among my cancer patients, and I suspect it holds true for other specialists in their medical fields and during the end-of-life experience.

Simply stated, the faulty message was this: Because you are responsible for your health and wellness, and because attitude is important in your well-being, if your cancer progresses or if treatment is ineffective, this clearly means you are not trying hard enough. Somehow, it's your fault if the cancer progresses. This is simply not true.

By placing the responsibility for survival on the patients and ignoring the fact that cancer and other diseases are also bio-logical processes—and patients don't have control over such phenomena—these faulty messages create a dark downside. It's not a matter of fighting hard enough or losing the battle with cancer. Certain things are simply beyond the control of human beings, patients and doctors alike.

That said, the importance of attitude and disposition cannot be discounted. And these can make a huge difference—for better or worse—in terms of quality of life and well-being in end-stage patients.

Pain of the Soul

Without question, an overwhelming proportion of dying patients—perhaps even more than half—have significant pain, even though there has been tremendous awareness of this phenomenon in the medical community. Dr. Eric Cassell, a renowned thinker on healing and suffering, described suffering as equivalent to the notion of total pain, which involves a phys-ical, social, psychological, and spiritual dimension.

We in palliative care are hopefully more attuned to the multifaceted dimension of suffering in patients. I want to think we have a sensitivity to inquire of patients about their needs over and above the pain caused by cancer, heart disease, or some other situation.

We are learning from social scientists and the clergy and the psychological community that meaning and purpose are absolutely crucial for a state of well-being. The terminally ill patient does not contribute to society as they once normally did, so there needs to be a shift to seek meaning and purpose in other ways. Although patients are obviously concerned about having their pain relieved, they also need a sense of control in their environment.

My medical colleagues and I recognize that during the dying process, the patient is wrapped in an envelope of losses: physical and cognitive losses, social and emotional losses, and also a spiritual loss bringing into question their faith or belief system.

We've also learned that there is the "work of grief," where patients need to process and evolve through accepting the reality of the loss of health, experiencing the pain of their loss and embracing that reality, and recognizing that family members will grieve the deceased partner or spouse or parent or sibling who is no longer available, necessitating an emotional relocation.

These are the tasks of grief that the community in general and individuals specifically must work through. One wise clinician commented that the only way to get over grief is to go through it. This is a process that cannot be fast-forwarded; nor can it be made better with a pill, a patch, or some short psychiatric intervention. (I am a fan of longer-term grief counseling, though.)

There is increasing recognition about spiritual pain where individuals question their previously held belief system. Almost all patients verbalize the sense of regret and despair and hopelessness when faced with a life-threatening or life-disabling illness.

I always go back to the words of that wise chaplain who, as I mentioned earlier, defined spirituality as an inner search for meaning and purpose, especially when faced with times of chaos and uncertainty. There are multiple definitions of this term, but, to me, this has always seemed the most workable.

The healthcare team should be expected to engage the patient in these meaningful dialogues but also to recognize that there may be a role to bring on board the counselor who can help the patient.

There are now recognized guides to spiritual assessments, and asking such open-ended questions as "How are you doing?" "How are you handling this situation?" can open up a rich tapestry of dialogues. It is almost impossible for patients to embrace spiritual healing and a sense of serenity if physical signs and symptoms are not addressed.

If a patient is nauseated, vomiting, and racked with pain, it is certainly not reasonable to expect that patient to become intensely spiritual. One aspect of the palliative care toolbox is recognizing the importance of symptom control and providing a pathway for an in-depth appreciation of an existential spiritual crisis.

Occasionally, patients will ask the team for a hastened death by injection or by some other intervention. It's important to be "present" and to ask the patient why they are seeking this sort of intervention. In general, it is typically a concern about loss of meaning, purpose, and control.

Terminally ill patients are at risk for suicide and are at a higher risk than the general population. The older individual, especially Caucasian men who are widowed or living alone, are at five times higher risk for suicide than the general population.

It has been well recognized that there is a healing power to touch. There is also the power of presence in leading to a healing and comfortable environment. The act of simply showing up can dramatically impact a patient's well-being, as we have already seen.

So, in summary, we recognize that there are profound psychological and spiritual sources of pain and suffering, and the medical team and the family need to recognize that there are appropriate interventions to somehow ratchet down the intensity of suffering at the end of life.

Spirituality and Religion

In the clinical setting we commonly hear, "I am spiritual, but I am not religious," which means that the individual has a sense of the omnipotent but disavows a formal faith connection.

No matter the source of spirituality or formal religion, both have a place at the bedside for patients and families when confronted with the end-of-life reality.

In early May 2013, clinicians from major medical centers through the Harvard system published a fascinating study of several hundred patients who had advanced cancer. The authors clearly documented that patients who acknowledged significant spiritual support from religious communities were far more likely to embrace aggressive care at the end of life. These individuals were less likely to receive hospice care, more likely to die in an intensive care unit, and more likely to receive intensive life-sustaining interventions.

On the other hand, when patients perceived that there was substantial spiritual support from the medical team, there were far fewer aggressive interventions, fewer deaths in the intensive care unit, and a greater use of hospice.

So let me summarize the findings. The 340 patients receiving spiritual support from their communities did not embrace a de-escalation of care but really opted for aggressive interventions, such as the intensive care unit. On the other hand, when the spiritual support came from the medical team, patients were far more reasonable, willing to go down the road of hospice and stay out of the intensive care units. What sense can we make of this fascinating study?

Well, the authors very reasonably suggest that the members of the religious community cannot be expected to understand the nuances and the subtleties and the complexities of a patient's illness. A common belief from the religious communities would focus on the role of perseverance through hope—the role of suffering and the hope for a miraculous resolution or healing of the patient's illness. In other words, the religious community, in effect, is urging the patient to "hang in there" or "hold on" while we wait for some divine intervention.

On the other hand, the medical community would have a far more realistic understanding of the patient's reality, and we have a responsibility to outline for the patient and family the anticipated trajectory of aggressive care. When this is done in an appropriate manner, patients are far less willing to go down the road of aggressive therapies.

At the end of the day, what do these kinds of studies mean? One important take-home message is that patients need to clearly convey to the health community that they, the patients, embrace spirituality, and what it means to them; we on the provider side need to embrace and understand what this means to the patient and family so that a reasonable middle ground can be reached.

A clinical dilemma we commonly see, especially in the hospital, is the expectation that the patient will be cured of their disease or condition. The expectation that if the patient can be sustained "just for a little while longer," there will be some divine intervention. While we each hope for this event, we do have a responsibility to put this into a proper perspective.

Interestingly, the spiritual support I see is a spokesperson for the patient's faith community at the bedside interacting with a ritual service of prayer, rosary or prayer beads, incense, or some other ceremonial celebration of faith.

These affirmations of faith are of tremendous value in enhancing quality of life of these patients with complex conditions. However, with the religious communities, spiritual support was not associated with enhanced quality of life near death. This is a complex area. We cannot sit on the sidelines but must clearly have a meaningful dialogue of how to maximize quality of life, coupled with the patient's spiritual expectations.

Glass Half Full?

Another important issue that often arises among family members is whether their encouragement and support of the patient makes any difference. As mentioned, there has been an emerging interest in the role of attitude and disposition and how they impact dealing with cancer, specifically lung cancer.

Studies from the Mayo Clinic have identified several hundred patients who had previously taken the MMPI, the Minnesota Multiphasic Personality Inventory. This paper-and-pencil test has been acknowledged for decades as being valid and reliable. On the basis of established scoring norms, some patients were deemed to be optimists and some patients were deemed to be pessimists.

Over a number of years, some of these patients developed lung cancer, since it is such a common cancer. A number of investigators raised an important question. How did the optimists do, compared with pessimists? In a peer-reviewed, respected medical journal, a study found that individuals who had a pessimistic style (glass half empty) did far worse with their cancer than individuals who had a more optimistic view of their illness (glass half full).

This paper fulfilled all of the statistical requirements for validity and was of tremendous importance. The authors reasoned something like this: Let's suppose someone has an early-stage lung cancer, and that person is an optimist. By definition, that person will seek out appropriate medical care, will aggressively evaluate hospitals, doctors, and surgeons, and will vigorously pursue the best possible treatment. On the other hand, the pessimist, by definition, is not prone to do any of these things. This person will let nature take its course and will have a very bad outcome. The optimists in this particular study lived several years longer than the pessimists.

A companion study assessed a series of lung cancer patients and gave them a simple questionnaire where they rated their quality of life. Ten out of ten was as good as it could be, whereas zero or one out of ten was pretty miserable. To the astonishment of the investigators, this simple questionnaire dramatically predicted and identified long-term survivors.

Studies are interesting, but what do these findings have to do with hospice and palliative care? These papers clearly document that if such symptoms as pain, shortness of breath, nausea, or vomiting are controlled, those patients will live longer than if the symptoms are not recognized. Let me explain.

Another study from the Harvard system examined several hundred patients who had lung cancer. Each received a standard chemotherapy program, and half of the group were randomly allocated to a palliative care approach involving board-certified palliative care specialists. In other words, every patient had standard chemotherapy and half also had aggressive palliative care. To the amazement of the authors, the patients receiving standard chemotherapy plus palliative care survived almost three months longer than the patients getting only chemotherapy.

This was a groundbreaking study, and the American Society for Clinical Oncology has now gone on record as stating that palliative care should be incorporated into the standard management of patients with advanced cancer.

So we are now learning from peer-reviewed journals and appropriate statistical analysis that when symptoms are controlled, patients not only have a better quality of life but they also live longer, as opposed to individuals whose symptoms are not controlled—even in situations involving end-of-life care.

Grief in the Survivors

Clearly, patients grieve as life ebbs away, but another important dimension of the dying process is the grieving that the family experiences. A phenomenon that we commonly see in the hospital is that of anticipatory grief. So what does this mean?

It means that the family is getting ready for that final event where the patient will no longer be with us. And if they do not recognize this phenomenon, they can experience great stress and frustration. With anticipatory grief, families demonstrate mourning (an inner feeling of meaninglessness) and at the same time act as if the patient has already died. They might talk about the patient in the past tense. I see this every day.

Grief takes emotional and physical work. Some tasks of grief that families might undertake are these:

- Accept the reality of the loss. This means that the health and the vitality and the energy of the patient are drifting away. And if the patient has actually died, this is a final event from which there is no return.

- There are no shortcuts. There is no quick fix. Sedatives, medications, and sleeping pills delay the healing process and in most circumstances are not recommended for grieving family members.

- Family members, especially spouses, must adapt to an environment where the deceased is no longer present. This is a painful and intense experience. Adaptation is a process, and it takes time. The community and some family members quickly forget. Life goes on. And the bereaved are left in a limbo land from which some never recover without loving support and sometimes professional guidance.

- Emotionally adjusting to a life without the deceased and carving out meaning and purpose in a world, either as a single person bereft of a partner or as an individual without that child or parent or sibling who meant so much, can be incredibly painful and incredibly lonely. In terms of losing a spouse, in general, we are a society of couples, so this presents its own challenges. In terms of other loved ones, every individual feels the pain of loss differently, but we all feel it. We are a society of connectedness, and so we must find ways to adjust to our "new normal."

In general, most of us do work through these devastating circumstances, but a minority of individuals never recover. There have been extensive studies about the four types of complicated grief, which I have summarized here:

1. **Chronic grief.** This is usually defined as overwhelming episodes of depression, anger, and guilt for six months after the death of the deceased.

2. **Delayed grief.** Years after an event, an individual may be overwhelmed by inadequate coping skills, anxiety, depression, and noncreative coping skills, such as risky behavior like drinking. A song. A restaurant. A smell. A holiday season can evoke overwhelming sadness and grief. Let me explain.

A distant relative in another city is a gentleman in his early forties. A very successful and prominent professional. He had a contentious, violent, emotional relationship with his mother, and following her death twenty years in the past, our relative never really addressed his feelings toward his mother. Recently, during Mother's Day, this individual had a complete meltdown. He could not function. Profoundly depressed, he became suicidal, and with intensive therapy and the input of credentialed mental health professionals, it became very clear that Mother's Day triggered a flood of emotions over a grief that was never resolved.

3. **Masked grief.** This refers to individuals who seem to outsiders to be absolutely cold and emotionless and aloof and detached relative to the death of a spouse, partner, or family member. Life goes on as if nothing happened. The day after the death is exactly the same as the day before the death. However, if these individuals do not come to grips with the reality of the loss, self-destructive behaviors, chemical dependency, and other coping mechanisms can become evident.

If grief and loss are not dealt with in a productive and creative manner, somehow, these feelings will come out in terms of physical illness, such as depression or anxiety, or in the form of some other spiritual sign of distress.

4. **Exaggerated grief.** This refers to activities and expressions that are over the top in dealing with the death of an individual. There are feelings of distraction. There is an inability to concentrate and an inability to form any sort of meaningful relationships. Thoughts of suicide become rampant. There are phobias and fears about illness and such benign situations as travel. These individuals need the help of credentialed and compassionate counselors and cannot be expected to simply "get over it" and move on with life.

The mind, the body, the spirit, and the soul are all interconnected. How we think and how we behave dramatically impact how we feel.

26
Who Cares for the Caregivers?

AT SOME POINT IN THE TRAJECTORY OF THE ILLNESS OF individuals at the end of life, important decisions must be made: For example, at what point should long-term care placement in a facility, such as a nursing home or hospice setting, be considered? Difficult decisions such as these tear the soul out of patients and families, but there does reach a point where, based upon family and social circumstances, the remaining caregiver is simply unable to shoulder the burden and that person's health continues to deteriorate in tandem with that of the person requiring the care.

Raye's father-in-law was in a near-vegetative state in a nursing home. He couldn't move; he didn't speak. How long could he live like this? Doctors kept saying maybe another month. Then another three months. Her mother-in-law drove to the nursing home every day. She fed her husband and attended to his needs. Every day. For three years.

His care had eaten up every dime of savings from his retirement plan and every monthly check from his pension. Raye's mother-in-law suffered what they suspected was a stroke. She spent time in the same nursing home as her husband and then regained enough function to move to assisted living, creating a real dilemma for the entire family. Such circumstances are not uncommon.

Caring for an individual with a serious or life-altering illness can take a devastating toll on the caregiver and also on other

family members. In the clinic and in the hospital, we repeatedly see caregivers exhausted, irritable, compromising their
own health, and not being able to function rationally in making
decisions for the patient.

With the shifts in the demographics of the American society
and with adult children often living far away from their parents,
it is the healthy spouse who often bears the burden of caregiving.
Sometimes, when adult children live nearby, it is the daughter
or even the daughter-in-law. Less often it is the son. What is the
lesson here? Have daughters? Seriously, the lesson is that families
need to have a plan that can be implemented to help both the
patient and the caregiver.

Caring for Yourself

The logic goes something like this: You must take care of
yourself if you are to be of use to your loved one who is dying. But
that's easier said than done when caregiving may have involved
years of care in the home, including all activities of daily living.

Caregiving outside the home may involve frequent trips to the
assisted living facility or nursing home or hospital. It may involve
other issues as well: Fighting with family members (especially
those out of town who aren't involved in the day-to-day care)
who have other ideas about care and outcomes. Paying bills,
arguing with billing offices, filling out tedious forms. Errands,
sitting by the bedside, watching pointless TV shows just for
something to take your mind off reality, endless doctor visits,
in and out of the car, worry, distressing late-night phone calls,
falls, ambulances—those who have been in this situation know
what I'm talking about.

Burnout among caregivers is a huge concern. Let me offer
some thoughts.

Regardless of the caregiver's age, there needs to be some focus
on physical fitness. Realistically, these individuals might not be

running a marathon, but they need to be encouraged within reason to walk at least thirty minutes a day, five days a week, either outside or on a treadmill. Alternatively, they can use a stair climber or an elliptical, or engage in some related activity, even walking up and down hallways in a nursing home or hospital. Typically, caregivers will claim that they don't have time, but we try to emphasize that if they don't have time now—or make the time now—they will certainly have plenty of time down the road when they will likely be impaired.

We also stress the importance of some form of resistance work either through bands, machines, or free weights. There are some data that starting at age thirty we lose approximately 1 percent of our muscle mass and strength per year. So, over the course of many decades, the unfit individual will basically give up or compromise one-third of their muscle mass. Those are muscles they may need to lift a loved one out of bed or assist them to get up from a chair.

There also needs to be some attention to the daily routines of life. Without having a list of priorities, without writing things down, and without having some schedule and some structure to the day, life can simply become a joyless grind.

Caregivers must understand that they cannot multitask. They cannot do two things at once, and to be scanning email, signing documents, and listening on the telephone is an absolute recipe for disaster, especially when there is a responsibility for someone who's so acutely ill.

Another dimension of this healing environment is that of connectedness and community. It is crystal clear that the caregiver who is isolated and marginalized is at a profound risk for all sorts of physical and emotional issues. Support groups, church and belief system gatherings, and community support are absolutely vital in order to go the distance in dealing with some difficult situations.

Yoga and meditation classes provide not only community and connectedness but also a spiritual dimension that has no religious affiliation. Even a quiet twenty-minute visit to the hospital's chapel can help turn off the head chatter and bring peace.

On a practical note, here are some suggestions for caregivers on managing the day-to-day tasks that come with the job:

- Assign jobs to family members and play to their strengths. If a sister-in-law is good with paperwork, let her handle the huge pile of medical bills and mail from the insurance company, Medicare, and so on. If a niece is a critical care nurse, have her research any medical issues or develop questions to ask at the family meeting with care providers. The accountant nephew can fill out forms and monitor finances. The teenage computer wizard can do private family posts and handle email updates.

- If Dad is the primary caregiver and has been at Mom's bedside for endless hours, give him a break. Take him out for a meal or offer him a night's sleep away from caregiving. Give him the relief he needs and feels confident accepting, knowing a competent person is there in his place.

- When well-meaning friends and neighbors say, "Just let me know what I can do," don't dismiss their offer. Take them up on it. Give them a job: mow the lawn, feed the dog, wash the laundry, bake a pie, pick up pizza, call the minister, drop this at the post office, pick up a few items at the grocery store.

- Make sure the primary caregiver has power of attorney to write checks from the ill family member's account so that bills are paid on time and without penalty.

- Keep a three-ring binder of essential documents so that no one has to scramble for them if the ill family member is switched to a different facility or provider. Include the advance directive, the healthcare power of attorney documents, the financial power of attorney appointment, the will, social security card, insurance cards, driver's license, veteran's information, medical history, prepaid funeral agreement and contact information for the funeral home, and any other pertinent documents. You can even take photos of some of these and keep them on your smartphone. The efficiency of having key documents on hand helps to keep stress levels lower.

- Have a list of phone numbers and emails for all family members and friends who need updates. Again, the smartphone can help organize these numbers.

- Instead of making endless calls or texts, consider using an online website, such as Caring Bridge, to post updates on the loved one's condition. Some people find it comforting to be able to share their grief. Others find it annoying and prefer privacy. Facebook is probably not the best way to share information like this, unless you're careful about your privacy settings.

- Read helpful books on death and dying. I have listed some in the resources section at the back of this book.

How Palliative and Hospice Care Benefit the Caregiver

Palliative and hospice care benefit more than the patient. And this surprising finding is bolstered by two major studies showing that high-quality end-of-life care for patients also benefits spouses.

A national study conducted by researchers at Mount Sinai Medical Center found that spouses of patients receiving hospice care reported less depression, compared with surviving spouses of patients in similar situations who did not receive hospice. This study was in *JAMA Internal Medicine.*

Dartmouth investigators found that early palliative care for cancer patients reduced the stress burden on caregivers during the last month of the patients' lives. This study was in the *Journal of Clinical Oncology.*

In every case, the palliative care team and adult children should be aware of the high-risk individual for complicated grief. Conjugal bereavement is the loss of a spouse/partner, and this can have devastating consequences for the surviving partner, especially the male.

Without doubt, it is also clear that if depression is not addressed, there are dire consequences in terms of a decrease in quality of life and, equally important, a decreased life-span. By definition, a "major depression" is diagnosed if the condition has lasted for two or more weeks for most of the day, with symptoms including depressed mood, lack of interest in activities that once brought joy, indecision, and especially feelings of hopelessness and worthlessness.

These are signs and symptoms that should alert family members to the need for intervention.

So how can the family be engaged in managing depression? Without question, the intervention of a skillful therapist is obviously crucial. In some hospice organizations, social workers reach out to families by mail, email, and phone for up to a year or more after the loss of a loved one. These are times to grasp the extended hand and receive emotional support and a referral to professional help. Some hospices organize grief support groups, as do some funeral homes.

The input of other professionals, such as the clergy, may be appropriate unless the caregiver is a nonbeliever and would find religious intervention upsetting.

The family physician can address the medical side of depression. The appropriate use of antidepressant medications called

SSRIs certainly are indicated for some individuals. The usual antidepressants may take six to eight weeks to maximize their effect, so be aware of this ramp-up period.

We cannot ignore for a moment the profound psychological stress on the family, in particular, the primary caregiver. These individuals can be under crippling pressure from sleep deprivation and expectations that are often magnified by financial worries. About a third of families lose substantial savings while caring for someone at the end of life.

Bottom line: Caregivers can get absolutely overwhelmed with compassion fatigue, which is typically characterized by sleeplessness and the inability to make a decision. They can develop an overwhelming feeling of isolation, with little recognition for the work that they do. Most are never given permission to get that massage or manicure, play tennis, get their hair done, have a few hours to themselves. They need to understand that they are dealing not only with overwhelmingly complex medical decisions but also the nitty-gritty of life: insurance policies, income taxes, user names and passwords, legal issues, paying bills, home maintenance, juggling dwindling funds, among many other issues.

Life and death each takes their course. At some point, the job of caregiver is over. Certainly, that caregiver may also be the funeral planner and executor of the estate, and a whole new set of responsibilities will begin. Throughout every stage of the dying process and its aftermath, the caregiver needs continuing help to adjust to the new normal of life. This is paramount for physical, mental, emotional, psychological, and spiritual well-being.

27

What If the Doctors Ask about an Autopsy?

JANET DIED RELATIVELY YOUNG, AT FIFTY-FIVE, OF AN unspecified brain disorder. During her yearlong struggle for a definitive diagnosis, she had numerous brain scans and multiple hospitalizations, suffering brain bleeds and loss of function. Nevertheless, doctors just couldn't pinpoint the problem, only speculate that it was some sort of neurological disorder. But what?

Her family struggled with understanding why medical science could offer no answers during her lifetime. And in death, they were asked if they wanted an autopsy to perhaps find out.

The issue was one of uncovering important pieces of medical data for the family to know relative to their own health and well-being. Her two children and their children would benefit from the information. If it wasn't an inherited condition, they would be relieved, of course. If it were, they would lower the bar on any early symptoms.

So an autopsy was offered, and the family agreed.

Despite sophisticated imaging with PET scans and MRI scans and CT scans during life, which offered no answers for Janet, the autopsy at death can often provide valuable information for surviving family members and for medical science as well.

Autopsies today can be done with great discretion, and usually there is no cost. Rarely do they delay the funeral, and, to reiterate, they can often uncover important pieces of medical information.

For example, I recall one circumstance in which the autopsy found evidence of a dormant variety of tuberculosis, which put the family at risk unless treated. In another case, the pathology found a rare abnormality of the coronary arteries that could trigger sudden death (the patient had died of something other than heart disease). The family was alerted about this genetic possibility.

Most often, it is the medical staff that requests an autopsy (it's rare for the family to ask). Families often agree to the investigation, but we're seeing fewer autopsies now that families think scans during life can reveal all that is necessary to know. They often say this: "Dad has suffered enough. Let's not torture him anymore."

Sometimes, as in Janet's case, the autopsy offered no new clues as to the diagnosis.

Organ Donation

Let me mention organ donation. Organ donation in end-of-life situations involving age and/or chronic conditions is usually not encouraged simply because, by definition, these patients are critically ill (regardless of age), and their organs have experienced significant trauma, especially from decreased blood flow.

Organ donation, other than eyes or tissue, actually cannot be done if the patient dies outside the hospital, because of the need for life support until the organs are removed.

Some patients, however, donate their remains to a medical school for anatomical purposes in teaching. I applaud them. This is the type of information to include in your advance directive and arrange ahead of time with the recipient institution.

That said, I'd like you to meet Jessie. She opened doors for me in medical school in 1966. She was an African American woman who died of a drug overdose in her late thirties. She was my cadaver, and I got to know her more intimately than I have ever known any other human on earth. I continue to remain grateful to her and to her family for the generous gift of her entire body to further my study of medical science.

If you've ever been to a memorial service for people who have donated their bodies, you would have heard the poignant words from medical students who are grateful to the donor and the donor's family. This gift is truly unselfish. It will help an innumerable number of people in the future, making it a gift of inestimable value as well.

28

How Do We Plan for the Funeral?

DISCUSSING A FUNERAL ISN'T THE MOST APPETIZING OF FAMILY dinner table conversations, but maybe it should be. Some people plan their own services, right down to selecting the clergy, the speakers, the religious or secular passages to be read, the flowers, and the music. What a gift for their families.

For us on the palliative team, it's not unusual to discuss the funeral with a dying patient. Certainly, I have heard these discussions at the bedside, and I applaud families for making these final arrangements.

When someone is dying, unless they specifically choose not to discuss the funeral and burial arrangements—whether casket and internment, or cremation (urn or disposition of the ashes)—then such subjects are almost essential. Those with foresight may already have prepaid arrangements, which makes things that much easier for an already grieving family.

Under most circumstances, it is difficult for patients and families to discuss the specifics of the funeral. But being involved with patients and family members during this painful situation, I have witnessed some incredibly moving and powerful testimonials to the deceased. Sadly, I've also seen some social spectacles that were almost like a circus environment rather than an appropriate tribute to the deceased.

Some of the services that seemed the most poignant and relevant involved a limited number of speakers acknowledging the individual the person was during their lifetime. Equally important was each speaker's acknowledgment as to who they were and how they were related to the patient.

Some of the most memorable services included brief commentaries by selected family members. In one particularly impressive circumstance, a family spokesperson was agreed upon by the family to speak on their behalf. This was eloquent, appropriate, moving, and an important dimension to the healing process for those in attendance.

So how do we summarize a bewildering amount of information that is laced with sadness and despair and hope and renewal? What can we learn from the individuals who have fought the good fight, who have gone the distance, who have given it their best shot, and who finally acknowledge that life is not always fair, the good guys don't always win, and, ultimately, we all leave this earthly planet?

The memorable individuals had a number of characteristics that I have learned from and will share with you here:

- They valued the relationships in their lives—their friends, their family, their community, and their engagements with the people they cherished.

- They accepted early in the course of their disease that this was not a fixable problem. They also accepted that the treatments and the interventions and the technologies, in some settings, were worse than the condition itself. When that was the case, they opted to spend their energy on quality of life for the time remaining, making the end a softer and more grace-filled transition.

- They learned the concept of mindfulness, a focusing on each moment and each relationship with riveted attentiveness.

- They recognized that any decision that they would make would have far-reaching implications, not only for themselves but also for their family.

- Most memorably, these patients do not let their illness consume them. They are not particularly focused on the next CT scan but, rather, on other people and their welfare. This included those of us on the medical team.

29

Has Anyone Considered the Cost of Dying?

EACH DAY, I SEE THE SPIRITUAL AND THE PHYSICAL DEVASTATION of advanced illness. Unfortunately, another dimension of this tragedy that we cannot ignore is the economic reality of dying. I have mentioned costs as part of other discussions, but much of it bears repeating here in this analysis of financial issues.

Over the decades, I have seen many, many patients kept alive mechanically with tubes and technology, while their hearts failed, their livers and kidneys failed, and their brains withered away. Most families make prudent decisions once they are appropriately counseled about the futility of continuing these measures.

Some families, however, cannot face the reality of the dire situation. No one wants to make a decision to discontinue heroic measures, and without advance directives for guidance, we in the medical community are obligated to do whatever it takes when a family refuses to accept any decrease in the intensity of care. Tragically, many of these patients languish for days.

One patient in particular, as I recall, died on day 202 of her time in the intensive care unit, leaving the devastated family to face the grim reality of the economics of medicine.

A typical day in an intensive care unit in most major medical centers can average approximately $15,000. Under some circumstances, the bill can easily be much higher. No patient's insurance ever covers dollar-for-dollar costs. If we do the math, we are looking at a price tag of several million dollars.

Now, at one time in history, we would never put a price tag on medical care, but this is a different era, and we need to have some sense of responsibility for the cost of dying.

In an ideal situation and in a perfect world, patients would die at home serenely, surrounded by a loving family and adoring pet, with the patient quietly passing away in the arms of their devoted spouse or life partner. However, the grim reality is somewhat different. Although more patients are dying at home, a substantial proportion of patients will spend at least some time in an intensive care unit in a hospital setting during their last month of life.

A typical scenario goes something like this. A patient has an advanced serious illness, whether it is cancer or heart, kidney, or lung disease. Patients will bounce back and forth between home, the nursing home, and the emergency room and clearly will have stays in the intensive care unit. This revolving door of inefficiency can often bankrupt the most responsible family, and approximately one-third of our patients become almost destitute because of expenses.

We who are or will be patients need to ask some important questions about financial realities. Obviously, we will not put a price on life and death, but the prudent consumer needs to understand the significance of the "sticker price" and what the insurance industry sugarcoats as out-of-pocket expenses.

I had this discussion with a woman whose husband had retired as a surgeon. He was a beloved, gifted technician revered by patients and peers. While visiting on the East Coast, he had a serious stroke-like illness and sought the input of a neurosurgeon there during this medical emergency. This neurosurgeon very appropriately recommended a lifesaving surgical procedure.

The patient's wife dutifully connected with her insurance company to be certain that the surgeon and the hospital were "in-network," with the expectation that a high proportion of the bill would be covered. Please sit down as I finish this story. Several weeks after hospital dismissal, the patient received a bill of $164,000. Yes, that figure is correct. And, frankly, it's rather low compared to some other nightmares I have heard about. The patient and the family went through the appropriate channels. How could this happen?

Well, it happened because the surgeon and the hospital, although in-network, requested the surgical operative room assistance of a head and neck surgeon, a plastic surgeon, and a vascular surgeon—none of whom were in-network. They were independent contractors who billed the patient separately. Moreover, the anesthesiologist was part of a private group even though the anesthesia group worked within the hospital, which was in-network.

So we have the perfect storm where the patient did all the right things—went through the appropriate channels—but did not understand how the game is played or how to have been a savvier consumer.

Now let's be fair. When faced with the need for lifesaving surgery, the last thing most of us think about are the insurance issues, but we need to be proactive or we will get a big surprise in terms of a big bill. And, certainly, while I am at the bedside of the patient, I do not know (or care) about who's paying for what and how much care costs. My care is not determined by the infamous "wallet biopsy," a term that describes whether the patient has insurance or means to pay.

We physicians often do not know how much a procedure costs or how much a medication costs or which doctors are in which insurance PPO or HMO network—although I do know that some FDA-approved cancer drugs cost as much as new cars, every month, and I'm talking about a Lexus.

Patients eligible for Medicare can often be dismissed from the hospital to an intermediate facility for rehabilitation or to a nursing home, and with certain qualifications, Medicare pays for the first 100 days. Never assume that Medicare will pick up the bill, however. So it is wise to schedule a sit-down meeting with a hospital or facility financial representative and ask questions and take notes.

The same is true if your loved one is in a hospice facility that operates on a per diem from Medicare. If the patient requires an emergency room visit or expensive treatments or interventions, that per diem is quickly exceeded, and the hospice goes into the red. So if that patient requests an emergency room evaluation, the family needs to understand that they may be responsible for the costs of that ER visit.

Let me explain why the higher the cost for care, the lower the quality of life for the patient and the lower the quality of death during the final weeks of life. These observations are from a study in the *Archives of Internal Medicine.*

Every day at the tertiary medical center (the highest level of hospital, usually a teaching hospital associated with a medical school), I see a subtle nuance that insists on aggressive, technology-driven therapies that have virtually no chance of helping patients who are terminally ill.

I see patients insisting on PET or CT scans when they are not medically indicated. High-tech intrusions, or yet another round of chemo, for many patients in dire circumstances are not necessary and can cause further harm. That's not what hope looks like. So, like the study on quality of life and death discovered, patients are subjected to more medical intervention (at their own insistence or because of poor medical advice) at the cost of their quality of death.

As our population ages and as the usual medical networks become less accessible and less user friendly, we are faced with the subtleties and the nuances of the economics of who lives, who dies, and who pays. Nothing compounds the tragedy of a loss more than opening the mail when the medical bills start coming in.

30

What Is the Role of Complementary and Alternative Medicine at the End of Life?

ONCE TRADITIONAL THERAPIES HAVE BEEN ABANDONED, THERE is overwhelming interest, curiosity, and hunger for alternative, complementary, and integrative therapies addressing the needs of people at the end of life. Some may have pursued these avenues during their traditional treatment as well.

Historically and traditionally, we in Western medicine have demanded randomized clinical trials with a placebo control to document the effectiveness of an intervention. However, it is now becoming clear that some therapies that enhance quality of life and sense of well-being do not lend themselves to a formal, randomized trial.

I'm talking about acupuncture, massage, prayer, meditation, and mindfulness. These practices clearly modulate the immune system and impact upon subtle chemicals secreted deep within the brain, which increase a sense of well-being.

These are some of life's mysteries that we just need to accept. For example, consider once again my explanation about the benefits of air gently blowing across a patient's face.

Aromatherapy, oils, and various derivations of massage, such as reiki, clearly have something to do with helping patients feel better.

Now, what about marijuana at the end of life? This is an area fraught with tremendous legal and medical controversy. Most states have clear indications for the use of medical marijuana, including treatment of autism or restless leg syndrome. In general, marijuana can be prescribed under selective circumstances and clearly may have a role in controlling anxiety and nausea. However, the definitive and generally accepted studies in this area have been subject to scrutiny and controversy.

Traditional Asian medicine focuses on the role of meridians, and there is evidence that pressure points in the wrist and in the hand have something to do with helping patients feel better.

I vividly remember an acupuncture exhibition at Mayo Clinic. The discussant was a prominent neurologist at the University of Minnesota. He showed a video from Southeast Asia where water buffalo and elephants had been disabled by an arthritic-type condition. They were treated with acupuncture—and, voilà!— they were back to work. This clearly is not psychosomatic or imaginative. No voodoo. Real.

Studies at Duke have assessed the impact of a spiritual/religious community in terms of sense of well-being. Individuals who are part of a formal church group have a better quality of life and an enhanced sense of well-being, compared to individuals who disavow any faith connection. It may well be that the power of the social support is a factor. However, any social group, even the bowling team or yoga circle, can be a source to provide social connectedness.

Building on the observations of Holocaust survivor and psychiatrist Viktor Frankl, our search for meaning and purpose in life takes us down the road to observing how the connected person fared better than an isolated individual. It is also clear that attitude creates reality. Among patients with lung cancer, the pessimist does less well than the optimist. Similarly, the individual who sees the glass as half full does better than the individual who sees the glass as half empty.

So we have learned that attitude creates reality (in an earlier discussion), and we do need to keep an open mind to some of these interventions.

A million years ago, humans sat around the campfire to ward off the winter cold and often reached down to pet a dog who became a faithful companion not only as a hunter but also as a protector. That relationship forged the animal/human bond, which has withstood the test of time. Petting the dog or stroking the cat releases a cascade of feel-good chemicals in our brains. Why not use this free medicine and bring the pet to the bedside of its dying master?

A word of caution: Patients come to us and report taking a bewildering array of supplements. They buy them at a corner drugstore or health food store or order them on the internet. Celebrities promoting lotions and potions are not experts. They are all in the money-making game. Buyer beware.

It's important that the healthcare team be aware of these additives. For example, high doses of certain vitamins can interfere with the blood-clotting mechanism and pose a great risk to a patient whose blood clotting we are trying to monitor at the end of life. Other supplements or herbs may contain harmful ingredients or no active ingredients at all.

We in the traditional medical model may not have all the answers, and if a patient chooses an intervention that appears to be safe—even though it has not withstood the test of a proven peer-reviewed article—we would be ill advised to discard it. Just tell us about it, and then we can discuss it.

31

What Lessons Have We Learned?

IF THIS BOOK COMES TO YOU WHILE YOU ARE SITTING AT THE bedside of someone you love—a mother, sister, father, brother, spouse, child, or friend—then you are surely distracted and emotionally drained. I have seen you in the hospitals.

These end-of-life journeys are never easy, even in the best of circumstances. But when life-and-death treatment decisions are being considered, the road is rough and filled with obstacles.

In these pages, I have tried to summarize forty years of bedside care with dying patients in hopes that my insights may provide comfort for you during these trying times.

If you have found that you didn't have the time or attention to read some of the preceding chapters—or if you just want a go-to spot for key issues that we have addressed—let me give you some bullet points to summarize the most salient aspects of our discussion:

- **Preferences.** When needing to make decisions about continuing certain courses of treatment or keeping a loved one on machines, ask the patient what they want. *Do you want to be on a dialysis machine to clean your blood of toxins because your kidneys are not able to? Do you want antibiotics and other medications to maintain your blood pressure? Would you prefer to die at home or in a hospice or under the light of a monitor in the intensive care unit? Do* your best to assure that you and the medical team know and carry out the patient's wishes, even if you don't agree with them. Wouldn't you want the same?

- **Comfort.** Know that most patients can be kept reasonably comfortable toward the end of life. However, we on the medical team cannot always manage delirium, agitation, and mental confusion. There is a fine line between keeping patients comfortable and alert and having them in a sleep-type state. Families need to understand that some patients simply cannot be kept pain-free and have them lucid at the same time. If family and friends need to be there "at the end" to tie up loose ends and say goodbye, don't wait.

- **Beliefs.** Rarely do we in the medical world ask about a patient's belief system, but this is absolutely crucial at end of life. In general, most patients are reassured when there is some discussion about their spirituality. To be clear, spirituality involves an inner search for meaning and purpose in the face of chaos and confusion. Religion, on the other hand, involves the rituals and mechanical procedures of a belief system. Insist that your medical team respect the beliefs and culture of the dying person.

- **Emotional well-being.** It is important to ask patients these questions: *What is it that keeps you up at night? What are you most concerned about?* The patient's concerns may be very different from those of the medical team or you as caregiver.

- **Life completion.** If the course of the disease state allows, patients want and need the opportunity to do the "final work": to talk about who they are, what they did, what they hope they achieved, what they wish they had accomplished, what they believe their legacy will be. Everyone wants to leave their mark on the world. Sometimes it's a loving family; sometimes it's a football stadium. If we don't ask them to tell us, we'll never know.

- **Treatment preferences.** Patients and families need to carefully understand the pros, cons, benefits, and expectations of treatment. At the end of life, treatment is almost never curative. Patients and families need to understand what they are "buying" from treatment. I remain astonished at the side effects that patients will tolerate, as well as the inconveniences to them and their families, for one chance in a thousand of some benefit from another harsh round of chemo or a mechanical heart device, which might extend life just a couple of miserable weeks. We on the medical team must ensure that patients and families have realistic expectations so that they understand all aspects of treatment and will be prepared to accept the inevitable.

- **Dignity.** Our humanity can sometimes be stripped from us in the intensive care unit. We are humans. We are each more than a clinical diagnosis. We are persons, each with a past and a future. Understand who the patient is, what work they did, what they are most proud of, and what they regret. I'd like to think that my medical colleagues would be more compassionate and ask about the patient's life story, but sometimes they need to be reminded by the family caregiver.

- **Quality of life.** Coupled with dignity, this involves giving the dying person a sense of well-being and psychological, emotional, social, and spiritual comfort. We often forget to ask, *What can we do for you?*

- **Family.** We need to be sensitive that the Hallmark card, the Norman Rockwell painting, the *Leave It to Beaver*, or *Ozzie and Harriet* family simply does not exist. Today, at the bedside, there may be second and third wives (or husbands), girlfriends (or boyfriends), life partners of the same gender, and all sorts of intricate relationships. Family need to be sensitive to everyone's needs. Recognize that with blended families and stepfamilies there can be great tension, especially when there are assets involved—and most especially when estate planning has not been properly thought out.

- **Medical team.** The relationship with a healthcare provider is absolutely crucial. Today, the primary care doctor is rapidly disappearing, and in this setting, patients cannot identify their primary provider, especially in a critical-illness environment. Patients and families need to know which member of the medical team is in charge of their care. Who is the quarterback? To whom should they relate the issues and questions that arise? Just knowing who that person is and that they are accessible can make all the difference.

- **Thinking ahead.** Bottom line, we need to plan; we need to think ahead. We need to be certain that all the dots are connected—not only from a medical (and legal) standpoint, with an advance directive and a healthcare surrogate for decision-making, but also, and of equal importance, from a financial (and legal) perspective, in terms of funds and estate planning.

All that said, at the end of life, all that matters is that we gave it our best shot—no looking back—and recognize that our lives have had meaning and purpose through the souls we have touched, the wounds we have healed, and the fences we have mended.

Life is a journey. The dying process is the last segment of that journey, and death is simply the final moment. We are all travelers together on the journey of life and death. I wish you and your loved ones a peaceful farewell.

RESOURCES
Books

Susan Bodtke, MD, and Kathy Ligon, MD, *Hospice and Palliative Medicine Handbook: A Clinical Guide*

Hattie Bryant, *I'll Have It My Way: Taking Control of End-of-Life Decisions*

Ira Byock, *The Four Things That Matter Most: A Book about Living*

Viktor Frankl, *Man's Search for Meaning*

Atul Gawande, *Being Mortal: Medicine and What Matters in the End*

Connie Goldman, *The Gifts of Caregiving: Stories of Hardship, Hope, and Healing*

Paul Kalanithi, *When Breath Becomes Air*

Elisabeth Kübler-Ross, *On Death and Dying: What the Dying Have to Teach Doctors, Nurses, Clergy, and Their Own Families*

Sherwin B. Nuland, *How We Die: Reflections on Life's Final Chapter*

Randy Pausch, *The Last Lecture*

Advance Directives

AARP offers downloadable forms for each state. Forms are provided by CaringInfo, a program of the National Hospice and Palliative Care organization, a national consumer engagement initiative to improve care at the end of life: *www.aarp. org/caregiving/financial-legal/free-printable-advance-directives/*.

End-of-Life Planning

The Conversation Project (*www.theconversationproject.org*) is a public engagement initiative with a goal to have every person's wishes for end-of-life care expressed and respected. The website contains free downloadable kits to start the conversation with loved ones.

ACKNOWLEDGMENTS

Not only am I grateful for forty-plus winters at Mayo Clinic and all the colleagues I have worked with over the years, I thank the tens of thousands of patients and their families for allowing me to share their life (and death) journeys—often in the face of life-threatening illness and gut-wrenching decisions. I will never forget the richness they brought to my professional life. I am humbled by their kindness and understanding.

Beverly Haynes, RN, the executive director of Seasons Hospice in Rochester, Minnesota, provided incredible insight into how hospice works in a stand-alone facility, which is truly a model of care for others. Her colleague Julie Assef, LSW, a social worker at Seasons Hospice, added rich detail to family interaction in a hospice setting. What I experienced in a hospital as a clinician was often far different from the more relaxed hospice setting. Beverly and Julie embody the best of the hospice caregiver.

I thank my colleagues in palliative care: Keith Swets, MD, MA, FACP, FAAHPM, HMDC, Associate Professor of Medicine and Section Chief, Palliative Care at the Birmingham (Alabama) VA Medical Center and Medical Director, Safe Harbor Palliative Care Unit, and Keith Mansel, MD, Professor of Medicine and Director of the Palliative and Supportive Care Services at the University of Mississippi Medical Center. They held my feet to the fire by reviewing the manuscript for medical accuracy, and, although I admit any remaining errors are still mine, I think they relished the task. It takes a certain type of human being to do what we do, day in and day out, and these two physicians are among the finest in our palliative field.

My administrative assistant, Candy Kostelec, has been supportive beyond measure. I am grateful for Candy's researching relevant scientific articles and, especially, for her loyalty (and putting up with my quirks).

Every author relies on early readers to keep him on task and act as a sounding board, and mine were diligent and honest. Special thanks to Fred Knight and Donna Miesbach. For sharing stories and allowing us to tell them here, I thank Candy Wood Lindley (who holds a special place in my heart as one of the most inspirational patients a doctor could ever know and whose own medical miracle remains just that). Thanks also to Rick Wollman, Judy Argintean, Richard Block, Julian Adair, Judy Batten, and Erin Brenner.

I thank Lisa Drucker, whose editorial red pencil kept us from coloring outside the grammatical and stylistic lines and whose judgment about choosing just the right words was, as always, dazzling.

To the book production team at Concierge Marketing, my thanks for your guidance and creativity, once again.

I thank my coauthor, Sandra Wendel, whose editorial brilliance and keen insights into the craft of writing were crucial catalysts to bring to the printed page our clinical experiences. Sandra's own experiences dealing with terminal illness in family members were powerful additions to our efforts.

And, finally, I thank my family: my wife, Peggy Menzel, and our menagerie of rescue and therapy animals, and my three sons and their wives and my two incredible grandchildren. Peggy patiently and tirelessly brought a sensitive touch to cold prose and knows the pain of dealing with the dying process of loving parents. Without my family's love and support, this story from the soul would never have emerged.

We've all heard the wise words telling us that it takes a village to raise a child, and no person is an island. This is so true that no book is forged without an armada of brilliant, creative pilgrims.

In the case of this book, there were other brave pilgrims, sufferers with one goal: to teach us how to live and to teach us how to die with peace and dignity.

Index

A

acupuncture, 240. *See also* alternative medicine
advance directive, 173–189
  do not resuscitate, 151–154
  download forms, 250
  life support, 168
  principles, 30–31
  right to die cases, 29–31
  right to refuse treatment, 32
  sample wording, 186–189
  where to keep, 175–176, 185
alternative medicine, 130
  aromatherapy, 159, 239
  healing power of pets, 241
  massage, 159, 239
  role at end of life, 239–241
Alzheimer's disease. *See* dementia
autopsy, 227–229

B

brain death, 15–16
burnout, 220

C

cancer, 51, 57, 78
  attitude, 205–208
  chemotherapy, 70, 108, 138
  cultural beliefs about, 43
  pain, 119
catheter, 137
capacity versus competence, 83–87, 95, 173–174
caregiver, family, 219–225. See also family
  outside caregivers, 196–197
  self–care for, 220–225
  survivor grief, 205–217
chemotherapy. *See* cancer
code status, 68–69. *See also* CPR and DNR
comfort care. *See* palliative care and hospice
complementary medicine. *See* alternative medicine
congestive heart failure, 143–146

constipation, 125, 131
COPD, 50, 149–150
CPR, 69, 151–152. *See also* DNR
Creagan, Edward T.
  board–certification in palliative care, 57–62
  family story, 34–40
cultural beliefs about death, 25–27, 244
  in conversations with a patient, 43

D

death and dying
  brain death, 15–16
  comfort measures at the bedside, 11
  cost of, 235–238
  definition of, 15–27
  helpful books about, 223, 249 (Resources)
  moment of, 12
  permission to die, 19
  process of, 8–11, 20–23
  pronouncing death, 17
  quality of life, 23–25
  right to die, 30–32
death rattle, 7, 9, 24
deathbed confessions, 155–165. *See also* family, secrets
defibrillator, 145
dementia, 78, 95
  agitation, 147–148
  as cause of death, 147
  at end of life, 146–149
  FAST score to assess, 147
DNR, do not resuscitate, 69, 151–154. *See also* advance directive and CPR
dying. *See* death and dying.

E

emphysema. *See* COPD
end of life. *See also* death and dying
  "good death" definition, 3–5
  family discussion, 82. *See also* family

moment of death, 12
role of palliative and hospice
care, 75–87. *See also* palliative
care and hospice
estate planning, 161–163
ethical dilemmas at end of life, 16.
See also physician–assisted
suicide
advance directive, 173–189
capacity versus competence,
83–87, 95
cultural beliefs about death,
25–27
optimism by physician, 51–55,
77
right to die, 29–32
use of opioids, 128
when is someone considered
dead, 16
with dementia, 148
euthanasia. *See* physician–assisted
suicide

F

family, family caregiver(s). *See also*
caregiver
assigning tasks, 222–223
bedside conversations,
158–161
bedside vigil, 19, 25, 158–160
conversations with the medical
team, 41–45
discuss end-of-life care, 82
hospice at home, 91. *See also*
hospice
life story at end of life, 37
making amends, 9
meetings, role of, 95–105,
110–112
reconciliation, 19
secrets, 73, 156
tying up loose ends, 17–19
unwelcome visitors, 197–198
when doctors deliver bad
news, 41–45
when family members don't
agree on treatment, 98–103
when to make a final visit,
9–10
feeding tube, 21–22, 111, 136
in an advance directive, 187

with dementia, 148
final wishes, 17. *See* advance
directive
funeral planning, 231–233

G

grief, grieving, 205–217
coping with, 215–216, 223–225
grief counseling, 209–210
types of, 215–217

H

healthcare proxy (healthcare
surrogate, healthcare power of
attorney), 17, 153, 170, 173–
189. *See also* advance directive
overriding patient's wishes, 181
hearing, sense of, during dying
process, 11
heart disease, 50, 60, 78, 112
as cause of death, 144
deactivating devices at end of
life, 145
LVAD, 144–145
home care companies, 196–197
home healthcare, 69, 137
hospice. *See also* palliative care
benefits for caregivers,
223–225
definition, 66, 89–94
diagnoses for admittance,
78–79, 90
difference between palliative
care and hospice, 66–67
history of, 77
levels of care, 80–81
Medicare benefit eligibility,
66, 78–81, 89, 103. *See also*
Medicare hospice benefit
settings, at home, 80–81, 91,
104; inpatient care, 81; nursing
home, 80–81, 92; residential,
81, 92, 104; respite care, 81
when to consider, 103–105

I

insurance coverage, 192–195. *See
also* Medicare hospice benefit
intubation. *See* respirator

K

kidney failure/dialysis, 85–86

L

life support. *See* respirator
living will. *See* advance directive
longevity, questions about, 47–55,
    90

M

marijuana, role at end of life, 240
Medicare hospice benefit, 66,
    78–81, 89, 103, 238. *See also*
    hospice
    eligibility for, 79
medication. *See also* pain and
    symptoms
    addiction, 127–128
    management, 115–117
    side effects, constipation, 125,
    131; nausea and vomiting, 126;
    confusion, 126
    supplements and vitamins, 241
    specific medications:
        acetaminophen (Tylenol),
        122
        antidepressants, 130
        benzodiazepines, 134,
        144
        dexamethasone, 58
        fentanyl, 127
        furosemide (Lasix), 134
        haloperidol, 124, 140, 144
        hydrocodone, 122
        hydromorphone, 122
        ibuprofen (Advil), 122
        lorazepam (Ativan), 11,
        134, 140, 144
        megastrol acetate, 136
        methadone, 124
        methyphenidate
        (Ritalin), 130
        metoclopramide, 136
        morphine, 11, 24, 84,
        119–131, 133, 144, 202.
        See also pain
        olanzapine, 140
        oxycodone, 122
        prednisone, 58, 84, 129
        risperidone, 140
        steroids, 58, 84, 129–130
        when to stop, 22–23
morphine. *See* medication
myoclonus, jerking of arms and
    legs, 10, 126

N

nerve block, 129. *See also* pain

O

oncology. *See* cancer
organ donation, 228–229
outside caregivers, 196–197
oxygen, use of, 11, 134

P

pain, 119–131. *See also* medication
    addiction to pain medications,
    127–128
    breakthrough pain, 124
    intractable pain, 128–129
    levels of, 119–120
    management, 122–123
    medications for. *See*
    medication
    morphine use at end of life,
    10–11. *See also* medication
    narcotics and opioids. *See*
    medication
        symptoms of use, 10
    nerve block, 129
    nonverbal cues for, 147
    pain level, pain scale, 119–120
    pain patch, 124–125
    pain receptors, 121
    side effects of pain medication,
    125–127
    spiritual pain, 120–121
    withdrawal symptoms, 127
palliative care, definition, 63–73,
    76. *See also* hospice
    at end of life, 59,72–73, 89
    benefits for caregivers,
    223–225
    difference between palliative
    care and hospice, 66–67
    family meeting, 96–105. *See*
    also family
    history of, 59
    in longevity and symptom
    control, 214
    qualifications for practitioners,
    65–66, 71, 76
    quality of life, 23–25
    role of, 60–62
    when to bring in a palliative
    specialist, 70–73
    when to end treatment, 117
    when to start and stop

medication, 115–117
pets, at the end of life, 159
physical therapy, role at end of life,
    130, 138
physician-assisted suicide, 89,
    199–203
"pull the plug," 100, 165–172. *See
    also* respirator

Q

quality of life, 48–55, 58, 207, 245
    with palliative care, 70, 117
questions about length of life,
    47–55

R

religion, role in death, 206,
    211–213, 240, 244. *See also*
    spirituality
renal failure/dialysis. *See* kidney
    failure
respirator. *See also* "pull the plug"
    intubation, 16, 137, 152
    removing, 165–171
    with COPD, 150
right to die, 29–32. *See* ethical
    dilemmas at end of life

S

spirituality, 240, 244. *See also*
    religion
    and religion, 211–213
    existential crisis, 2
    in grief, 205–207
    phases of dying, 9, 24–25
suicide. *See* physician–assisted
    suicide
survival time, 47–55, 90, 214
symptoms, during end-of-life care,
    133–141. *See also* medication
    and pain
    anxiety, 134
    appetite, thirst, hunger, 11, 21,
    135–137
    blood clot, 23
    blue discoloration of hands,
    feet, 12
    bowel obstruction, 125, 139
    confusion, 140
    death rattle. *See* death rattle
    dehydration, 115, 140

delirium, 23, 140
fatigue, 20, 137–138
incontinence, 10, 137
myoclonus, jerking of arms
    and legs, 10, 126
nausea and vomiting, 23, 71,
    111, 126, 138–139
pain. *See* pain
peripheral neuropathy, 70–71
pneumonia, 22
shortness of breath, 11, 68, 84,
    with COPD, 149
sleep, lack of, 23, 141
speak, inability to, 137
suffocation, fear of , 73, 119,
    133–135, with COPD, 149
swallow, inability to, 135
weight loss, 135–137
management of symptoms, 61,
    68, 83–87, 133–141
        to boost longevity, 214
medications used to manage
    symptoms. *See* medication

V

ventilation. *See* respirator

W

wills. *See* estate planning

About the Authors

Edward T. Creagan, MD, FAAHPM, is a medical oncologist and hospice and palliative care specialist who practiced at the Mayo Clinic for more than forty Minnesota winters until his retirement from active medical practice in late 2018. He is professor emeritus of medical oncology at the Mayo Clinic Medical School where he held the endowed chair as the John and Roma Rouse Professor of Humanism in Medicine, and he is now Emeritus Professor of Humanism in Medicine and an Emeritus Consultant in Palliative Medicine there.

He was named Outstanding Educator from the Mayo Clinic School of Continuing Medical Education and has received the Distinguished Mayo Clinician Award—Mayo Clinic's highest honor. He completed an elected term as President of the Mayo Staff.

Dr. Creagan was the first Mayo Clinic consultant board certified in hospice and palliative medicine. He is also board certified in internal medicine and medical oncology.

Dr. Ed (as he is known) received his medical training at New York Medical College and earned graduate degrees in internal medicine and oncology at the University of Michigan and the National Cancer Institute before joining the staff at the Mayo Clinic in Rochester, Minnesota.

In 2015, he received the Ellis Island Medal for contributions of descendants of immigrants.

He is the author of over 500 scientific papers and has given more than 1,000 presentations throughout the world, including his home state of New Jersey.

As an accomplished speaker, his presentations to both professional and consumer audiences are notoriously funny yet filled with useful lifestyle information on such topics as the healing power of pets, preventing stress and burnout, and surviving retirement. His presentations have such appealing titles and motivational content as Dr. Ed's 8 Commandments for Living Well, How to Live Long Enough to Cash In Your 401(k), and How to Talk So Your Doctor Will Listen. He is available to speak to corporate, consumer, and medical groups and invites inquiries.

With coauthor Sandra Wendel, he is the author of the fully revised second edition of his triple award-winning book, *How Not to Be My Patient: A Physician's Secrets for Staying Healthy and Surviving Any Diagnosis* (*www.HowNotToBeMyPatient.com*). He is the editor of the book *Mayo Clinic on Healthy Aging*.

An avid marathoner and golfer, father of three sons, and grandfather of two grandsons, Dr. Creagan and his wife, Peggy, live with a rescue dog and two rescue cats in Rochester, Minnesota.

He tweets @EdwardCreagan and @AskDoctorEd and blogs on www.MayoClinic.com, Mayo Clinic's online website for consumer health information. Readers may contact Dr. Ed at *www.AskDoctorEd.com*.

Coauthor **Sandra Wendel** is a skilled nonfiction book editor who lives in Omaha, Nebraska. Contact her at *www.SandraWendel.com*.

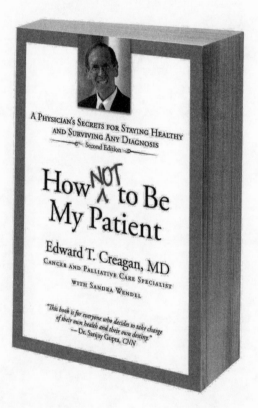

How ^NOT^ to Be My Patient

A Physician's Secrets for Staying Healthy and Surviving Any Diagnosis

Second Edition

Edward T. Creagan, M.D., F.A.A.H.P.M.

MAYO CLINIC MEDICAL ONCOLOGIST/CANCER SPECIALIST
AND PALLIATIVE CARE CONSULTANT
JOHN AND ROMA ROUSE PROFESSOR OF HUMANISM IN MEDICINE
PROFESSOR OF MEDICAL ONCOLOGY

WITH SANDRA WENDEL

WRITE ON INK
PUBLISHING

What others are saying about
How Not to Be My Patient

"I have shared the podium with my good friend Dr. Ed. The two of us—a cancer doc and a veterinarian, an unlikely tag team—understand the amazing healing power of the animal-human connection and have devoted our careers to this bond. I am delighted that, finally, medical doctors embrace the importance of our companion animals as a key part of the pet prescription. Dr. Ed explains this connection and devotes nearly a full chapter to the power of the 'Lab' results and 'cat' scan in modern medicine in his outstanding book about prevention and survival."

Marty Becker, D.V.M., Veterinary Correspondent
for the American Humane Association,
founding member of Core Team Oz for *The Dr. Oz Show*,
best-selling author and advocate for the healing power of pets

"Forget the TV doctors (please!). Dr. Ed Creagan is the real deal, a superb physician who knows what it takes for people to live long and well. In this book, he generously shares his experience and wisdom with the rest of us. I, for one, am taking his guidance to heart, and I hope to outlive him!"

Ira Byock, M.D., Professor, Geisel School of Medicine
at Dartmouth, palliative care physician, and
author of *Dying Well* and *The Best Care Possible*

"I saw Dr. Creagan at Mayo Clinic for a life-threatening condition thirty years ago. We looked at my prognosis and prayed, and then we got busy surviving. Sometimes the best medicine—besides a battalion of medical care—is a doctor who is kind, gracious, and understanding. That's Dr. Creagan. I thank God for His help, but I also thank Dr. Creagan for helping me survive a scary diagnosis. He says I'm a miracle. And I am."

Candy Wood Lindley,
author of *Face of Faith: Discovering a Different Kind of Makeover*

Introduction

We are each put on this planet
to do something that no one else can do quite as well as we can.

"He has cancer," they would whisper with pity and dread. The residents of my grandmother's rooming house would go to great lengths to avoid John G., the unemployed factory worker in room 212, as if somehow by just talking to him they would catch his horrible disease.

Most residents of 615 Hunterdon Street were down-and-outers, renting rooms by the day, week, or month. Most were unemployed, but a few worked at a neighboring bar called the PON, Pride of Newark (a sure contradiction in terms), if they weren't on the other side of the bar battling with the bottle.

Having cancer in 1952 was as close to a death sentence as awaiting the electric chair from prison's death row—perhaps faster. What we didn't know then about cancer could fill volumes. But for me, a precocious second-grader living with my Irish immigrant grandmother who owned the 22-room boarding house in the Ironbound section of Newark, New Jersey, being around someone with cancer was a defining moment—maybe not in medical history but in mine.

You see, the gentleman in room 212 had a colostomy, in which his bowels emptied into a bag on the outside of his body because colon cancer had destroyed part of his intestine. I was able to comfortably change his appliance (bag) and simply knew that I would care for people like this for the rest of my life. That was the way it was. No debate. No discussion. I just knew. This was my first experience with cancer. I was eight years old.

My first clinical encounter was as a second-year medical student at New York Medical College. The year was 1968. I was assigned an elderly woman with advanced cancer of the stomach. Sunken eyes, hollow cheeks, skin stretched over bare bones; she was a living cadaver. When I first walked onto the ward and saw her, I thought she was dead. But I found the courage to approach her bedside.

Who was this woman? Did she have a family? What made her laugh or cry? What biological nightmare brought her to this dismal fate? I found it intriguing—fascinating in a morbid way—that one cell went haywire, robbed her of her future, and eventually resulted in her death. She had no chance for a reprieve.

How did this happen? I was "hooked" on the journey to find answers to the cancer question. My classmates thought I was crazy to deliberately seek out the cancer patients. It was hopeless, they said. I was wasting my time and efforts. They were wrong.

A Disease of the Soul

I was initially attracted to the biology and the genetics of cancer and was intrigued with the notion of mixing various types of chemotherapy (chemicals used for treatment), then adding radiation and immune-related treatments. But it was soon obvious to me that my attraction was not a fascination with cancer as a disease of the body but cancer as a disease of the soul.

Over these past four decades, I have pursued a path chosen years earlier in a grungy rooming house helping a sick and sad old man. Through him and the 40,000 other encounters with cancer patients I've worked with at one of the world's foremost medical centers, I have discovered the majesty and the resiliency of the human spirit. I learn from my patients. I listen to their stories. And I learn to treat each day as a gift. A day not to be wasted.

In effect, the oncologist (the cancer specialist) becomes the spiritual leader—priest, minister, rabbi, for example—for patients and their families. I'd estimate that at least 70 percent of our time is spent simply listening to patients and hearing their stories, rather than dripping toxic chemicals into their bodies.

As a physician, I'm inspired to hear the survival skills and tactics of patients who are at risk of being crushed by life's unfairness. It is their 11th hour. And no governor is standing by on the hotline to commute their sentences. Those stories keep me going.

Every cancer patient is surrounded by a litany of emotional nightmares: the prodigal son who does not return; the wayward daughter who reluctantly returns home; the mortgage that is never paid off; the business reversals, shattered dreams, and missed opportunities (especially the chance to say, "I'm sorry" or "Forgive me").

The most painful words I hear far too often at the bedside are these: "I will never know how good I could have been. Maybe I could have made the big time, and now there is no time left." Yet, somehow, these patients continue to thrive and are a tremendous source of courage and admiration.

What I have learned from them is not to sweat the small stuff, but rather to savor each moment, to grasp it firmly, and to try to make the world a little better than it is right now. For me, each patient is a gift to be cherished.

We physicians need to understand that each patient is a person with a past and a present, a life spent dealing with a dreaded diagnosis.

Out of Suffering Comes Wisdom

The oncologist has "defining moments" every day if he or she takes the time to listen. Everybody has a drama. If we have patience, we doctors can come to know the human spirit.

We are each put on this planet to do something that no one else can do quite as well as we can. The lesson from thousands of patients is that everyone has a story. The overarching need of every human being is for recognition and acknowledgment. We want to be listened to, not preached at. We each say, in a special way, *Make me feel important. I am unique.*

Someone once said that everyone has at least one story good enough for a book, and perhaps this is mine. I wrote this book so that you can avoid cancer and other dreaded diseases. You have control over your destiny. You can and must take charge. As a patient, your job is to become the most empowered, the most knowledgeable person about your disease, because you are in charge of your decisions about treatment. No one has a greater stake in your health than you do. The buck stops with you, not your doctor.

"You're the doctor," some patients say to me, implying that I should advise them what to do. "No," I tell them. "You are the patient, you are in charge. Together, we will take this journey."

Sometimes, together, as doctor and patient, we may have to look at the relative futility of trying to treat advanced disease with current treatment plans. Many cancer treatments may worsen quality of life, and patients need to understand this reality. But let me be perfectly clear: For some cancers, and other diseases, the track record with current treatment is positive and hopeful and holds the potential for cure.

Let me share an amazing story. It was 1983. I had the privilege of evaluating a 56-year-old man for advanced lung cancer. He was referred to me from a prestigious medical institution in the Midwest. When I asked him what he was told about his illness there, he said, "They told me to pick out a good blue suit and six pallbearers."

He has returned to see me once a year every year since then. He has the same blue suit. Five of the six pallbearers are dead, and his original oncologist is in a nursing home. He always asks me how I am doing. Astonishing! He has lived with cancer, and he asks me how I'm doing!

This is what keeps us cancer specialists coming back.

How Not to Be My Patient

I inherited my father's fascination with the Sport of Kings— thoroughbred racing—and eagerly await the arrival of the Triple Crown. Most of us know the names of some of these three races: the Kentucky Derby, the greatest two minutes in sports; the Preakness; and the Belmont Stakes, the 1.5-mile route in New York that often signals the end of many thoroughbreds' careers.

I learned a lot at the track—far more than from any courses in sociology. The betting game comes with its own set of rules. The weekend gambler might just as well throw his money into the wind without some knowledge of the horses, the riders, the trainers, and the tracks. There is no such thing as luck. At the track we may lose money. The medical game is played the same way but with higher stakes. In medicine, we may lose our life or our quality of life.

Consumers of health care need to understand how the game is played. Medicine is at the crossroads. There are presently 79 million baby boomers marching in lockstep cadence into their 60s and 70s, who will place crushing pressures on the health care system during their older years. National changes with the Affordable Care Act on the health insurance side of the equation are evolving as we speak.

I am hardly a health care economist, but in the current climate the fees doctors get from Medicare do not fully cover the cost of providing the service. Mayo Clinic reports megamillion-dollar losses. Imagine the losses your medical clinic is taking. These deficits are not fiscally sustainable, so some health care organizations have limited their access for patients covered by Medicare. Some clinics have informed these patients that effective as of a certain date, they may be forced to pay cash for services.

Add those challenges to the issues patients face trying to get medical care. Sure, if you have crushing chest pain and go to the emergency room in a major metropolitan area, most likely you will get excellent care. But if you have a routine, nagging concern, you may have great frustration just getting an appointment.

You may not see a doctor but a "mid-level provider," such as a nurse-practitioner or physician assistant. Each plays an important role in medicine. However, the sands of time are shifting, and medical care, as we know it, is quickly fading from the scene.

We as patients need to understand the changing nature of medical students. Most are women, and it's highly unlikely that most of them will practice full-time. But now for the really serious news. About 95 percent of medical students are not going into primary care or general internal medicine or family medicine; they are specializing. So the boots are simply not on the ground to care for us when we have a problem.

Another part of this drama is much less publicized. Bureaucratic strangleholds on medicine and a bewildering number of regulations are driving physicians to retire at younger ages and at higher rates than ever before. If you doubt me, ask your doctor, especially if he or she is older than 50. Large numbers of patients need care. Fewer physicians are available to deliver care. And patients are bombarded with information on the Internet. What's a person to do?

Your Best Bet—The Daily Double

Here's the inside track. An ounce of prevention is still well worth a pound of treatment. As we head into an environment of cost containment and the ratcheting down of access to medical services, you need every scrap of sound medical information you can get to truly be in charge of your own health and longevity. Your best daily double against cancer and other serious diseases is still healthy lifestyle choices and early detection of disease. But there's much more.

Let's look at the odds: more patients flooding the exam rooms, a greater number of older patients putting pressure on a health care system with a dwindling number of doctors, regulations and low reimbursements from insurance programs forcing doctors to retire, and changes in the insurance and government program payments.

We as patients need to be savvy consumers because we will be buying our own coverage, and we need to understand what we need as patients and what we do not need. Marcus Welby, M.D., is no longer in practice, and we need to know how the game is played—or we lose. The best approach: stay fit, medically wise, and know your options because the "system" is still shaking out, and you can get lost and overwhelmed with life-and-death decisions.

Ideally, each patient and family has a primary care provider to be the medical quarterback. But less than 5 percent of medical school graduates enter primary care. All the other doctors in training are specializing. Why? I have connected with wonderful physicians in training over the last several decades. They are dedicated and compassionate; but they are concerned about lifestyle issues, and so they are less willing to have medicine become the primary life focus that it was for my generation who graduated medical school in the 1970s.

I vividly recall spending my days off in the emergency room of an inner-city hospital in New York in order to gain extra clinical experience. Few learners would do that today, and perhaps that is healthier.

Another issue: the primary care provider has more stress and burnout and less income than the specialists, so fewer learners enter this area of medicine. It's an economic, time-and-money decision.

I'm going to share with you how to make the best choices, the most important medical decisions, you will ever make in your life. And I'm not talking about track tips or stock tips. By the time I see most of my patients, they have weeks, not months, left to live. Let there be no doubt: They are courageous, and we have many, many success stories that defy what we know about cancer. But truth be known, about half of my patients never needed to walk into my exam room because their cancers were related to lifestyle choices they made along the way.

I'm not placing blame or guilt. There is little merit in looking back. I'm telling you the reality. The number 1 fear of the person on the street is not heart disease, AIDS, or arthritis. It is cancer. Public speaking is a close second, I am told. I can't tell you how to stand up in front of a crowd. But in this book, I will tell you what you can do, for yourself and your family, so you won't ever be my patient.

Although we cannot prevent all cancers and all scary diseases, we can place ourselves "on the rail," in a position to make the final sprint to the finish line. A guarantee? Of course not, but what I learned at my father's side at the track is that we can shift the odds in our favor if we have the knowledge to be proactive and involved in the most important race of our lives.

You can bet on it.